A Colour Atlas of
Adult Congenital Heart Disease

A Colour Atlas of
ADULT CONGENITAL HEART DISEASE

Leonard M. Shapiro
MD, MRCP
Consultant Cardiologist
Papworth and Addenbrookes Hospitals, Cambridge

Kim M. Fox
MD, FRCP
Consultant Cardiologist
National Heart Hospital, London

Wolfe Medical Publications Ltd

This book is one of the titles in the series of Wolfe Medical Atlases, a series
that brings together the world's largest systematic published collection of
diagnostic colour photographs.

For a full list of Atlases in the series, plus forthcoming titles and details of
our surgical, dental and veterinary Atlases, please write to Wolfe Medical
Publications Ltd, Brook House, 2-16 Torrington Place, London WC1E 7LT,
England.

CONTENTS

ACKNOWLEDGEMENTS

We are indebted to the many friends and colleagues who contributed illustrations for this text. In particular, we acknowledge all the physicians at the National Heart Hospital, past and present, who have looked after many of the patients illustrated in this book. We also wish to thank the following, who have lent us illustrations: Dr M Raphael, Dr M Rubens, Dr R Underwood, Dr D Longmore, Professor R Anderson, Dr E Olsen, Dr A Rickards, Dr Carole Warnes and Miss Caroline Westgate. The help of Miss Kathy Back in typing the text is gratefully acknowledged.

We would specifically like to thank Dr Jane Somerville, whose pioneering work in the care and management of many of the patients illustrated has made this book possible.

PREFACE

Minor congenital heart disease anomalies are common and serious congenital heart disease occurs in approximately 0.1 per cent of live births. The clinical picture of congenital heart disease has changed, particularly in the last decade, with the introduction of surgical operations which increase life expectancy in conditions which were previously fatal in infancy and childhood. Furthermore, the incidence of congenital heart disease is not falling (it is perhaps increasing) because more women with congenital heart disease are reaching child-bearing age and their children risk inheriting heart disease. In this atlas we deal with both minor and serious congenital heart anomalies. While it is impossible to be complete, we have attempted to describe the more important conditions.

Adult congenital heart disease is of importance to paediatric and adult cardiologists, general physicians and general practitioners, who are likely to see, and need to identify, not only the minor, relatively common conditions, but also those which are more serious. The pathology, physical signs and investigations of each condition are presented in order to demonstrate their anatomy and function.

There are very few books which deal with this complex subject and it is hoped that this illustrated format will help to make the subject easier.

Secundum atrial septal defect

Secundum atrial septal defect is a relatively common form of congenital heart disease, frequently associated with more complex forms of congenital heart disease. It is a defect of the secundum septum in the area of the fossa ovalis. Secundum atrial septal defect may occasionally be associated with inherited conditions, but almost half of all patients are asymptomatic and detected only on routine clinical examination. The characteristic clinical finding is a fixed splitting of the second heart sound throughout the respiratory cycle and the chest radiograph will show pulmonary plethora. Cross-sectional echocardiography can be used to visualize the defect directly and to detect associated abnormalities.

Most patients will undergo routine closure of an atrial septal defect as soon as the diagnosis is made, but in those patients who do not have surgery atrial tachyarrhythmias and right heart failure may occur in later life.

1 Macroscopic section of a secundum atrial septal defect, showing a moderate-sized defect, viewed from the left atrium.

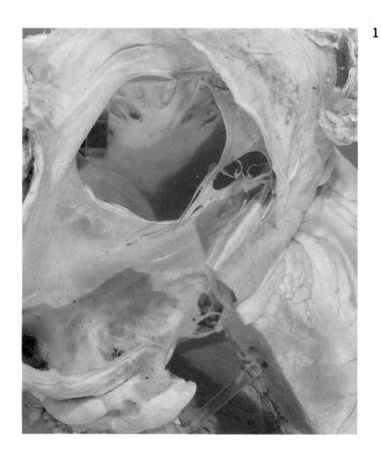

1

2

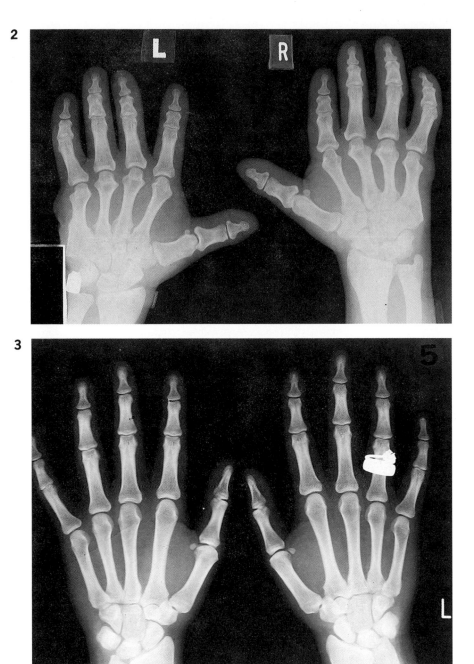

2, 3 Inherited conditions associated with secundum atrial septal defect include the Ellis-van Creveld syndrome (**2**) and the Holt-Oram syndrome (**3**). The Ellis-van Creveld syndrome is characterized by polydactyly of the hands, dwarfism and dysplasia of the fingernails. It is inherited as an autosomal recessive trait. The Holt-Oram syndrome has hypoplasia of the greater multi-angular carpal bone of the radial side, resulting in a small thumb on the same plane as the fingers. There is also a spectrum of upper limb abnormalities in which any of the upper limb bones may be absent, hypoplastic or deformed.

4, 5 The characteristic auscultatory abnormality of secundum atrial septal defect is fixed splitting throughout the respiratory cycle of the second heart sound frequently with an ejection systolic murmur (ESM). Often, particularly in large atrial septal defects, there will be a tricuspid flow murmur and a right ventricular third heart sound (arrowed)(**5**).

6 The electrocardiogram in secundum atrial septal defect will show right bundle branch block with the axis being towards the right. The rhythm in this example is sinus, but particularly in adults, atrial fibrillation and atrial flutter are common complications.

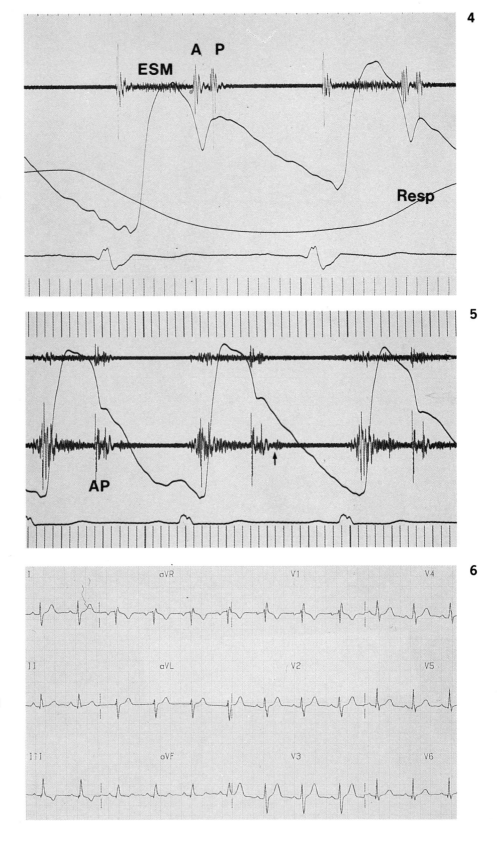

7

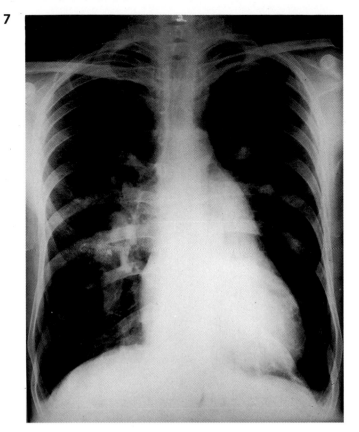

7, 8, 9 Chest radiograph in atrial septal defect will show a prominent pulmonary artery with pulmonary plethora (**7**). In cases where the shunt is large, the plethora will become increasingly obvious and in addition, cardiomegaly will develop (**8**). It is important to differentiate the dilated pulmonary artery, seen in atrial septal defect, from idiopathic dilatation of the pulmonary artery where there will not be evidence of pulmonary plethora (**9**).

8

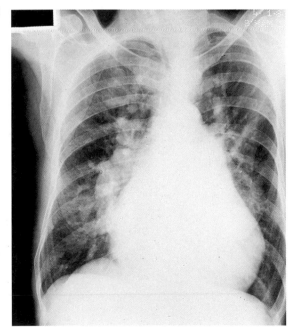

9

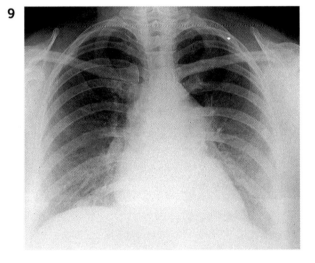

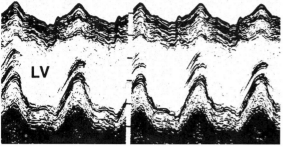

RV

LV

10—17 Echocardiography may be used to visualize the atrial septum directly or study the effect of right ventricular volume overload. Figure **10** shows the M-mode echocardiogram in an atrial septal defect with dilatation of the right ventricle (RV) and paradoxical septal motion. When imaging, using cross-sectional echocardiography, the subcostal view may be used to demonstrate the defect in inner-atrial septum (**11**). From the parasternal view, the position of the defect in the inner-atrial septum can be seen close to the aortic root (**12**) or lower (**13**)(arrowed). The apical view

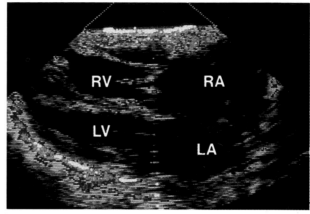

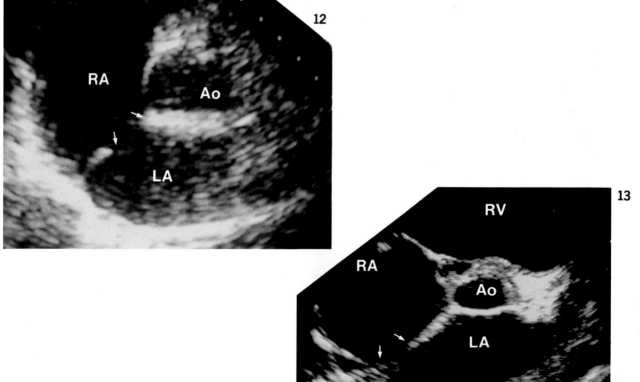

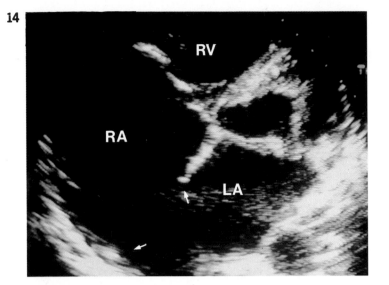

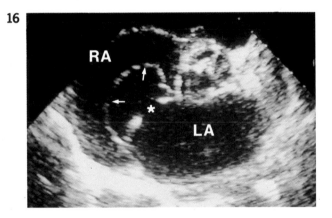

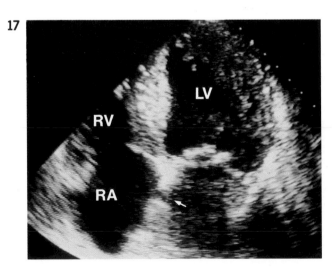

(14) may be used to show the size of the right ventricle and the movement of the inter-atrial septum during cardiac cycle. With right ventricular dilatation, the right atrium is also enlarged and the disparity between the size of the right and left atrium can be seen (14). Occasionally, a patent foramen ovale (15) may be seen by cross-sectional echocardiography and is an important differential diagnosis (arrows). Figure 16 shows an inter-atrial septal aneurysm bowing from the left to the right atrium (arrowed). This aneurysm moves with the cardiac cycle and may be a source of both emboli and atrial tachyarrhythmias. It has been suggested that such aneurysms represent a closing atrial septal defect (*) and in this example they are coincidental (16). When imaging the inter-atrial septum from the apex, the area of interest is perpendicular to the ultrasound beam and septal drop-out may occur, which simulates an atrial septal defect (17).

18 Colour flow Doppler echocardiograms (apical four chamber view) showing flow (arrowed) crossing the atrial septum (**a**), passing through the tricuspid valve (**b**) and into the right ventricle (**c**).

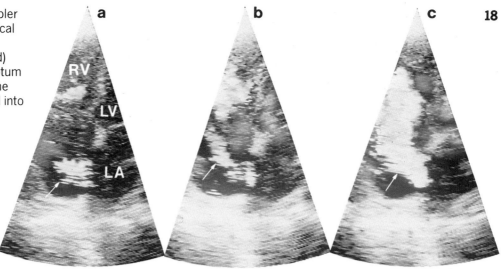

19 Using gated blood scanning it is possible to calculate the size of the shunt in atrial septal defect.

20—22 Magnetic resonance scans in secundum atrial septal defect will clearly delineate the anatomy. In this sequence of scans a dilated right atrium and right ventricle are evident (**20**), the inter-atrial septum and the defect (arrowed) can be seen (**21**) and the disparity between the dilated pulmonary artery and normal aorta can also be seen (**22**).

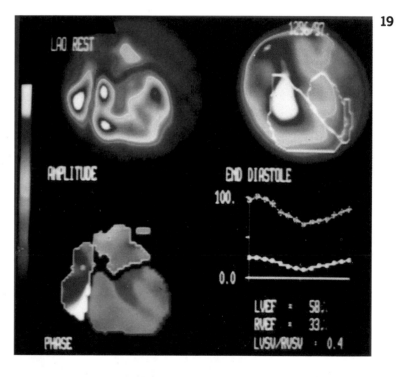

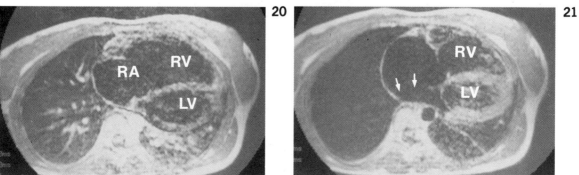

22

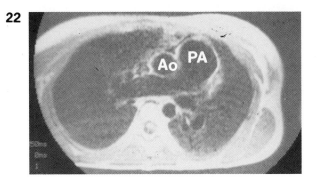

23

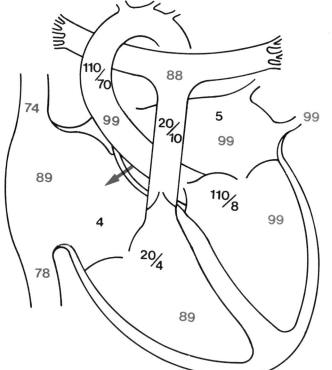

23 On cardiac catheterization a step-up in saturation will be present at atrial level with a left to right shunt of 2.2:1 and a normal pulmonary artery pressure.

24

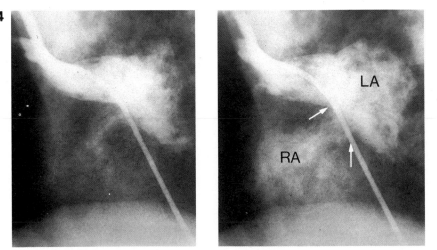

24 Pulmonary vein injection (left anterior oblique cranial projection) showing filling of the left atrium and contrast crossing the atrial septal defect into the right atrium.

25

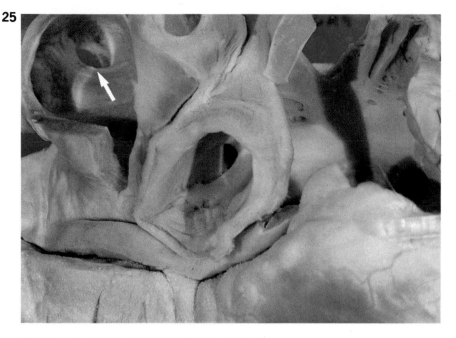

26

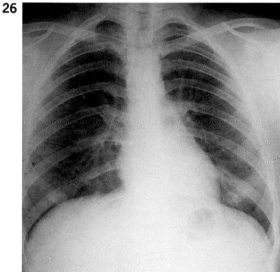

25, 26 Sinus venosus atrial septal defect is a form of secundum atrial septal defect in which the defect lies high in the septum so that the superior vena cava overrides it. Figure **25** shows a sinus venosus defect (arrowed) viewed from the atria; the relationship to the superior vena cava is evident. The sinus venosus defect may be recognized radiographically by the absence of the shadow of the superior vena cava high on the right side (though the vessel is usually shifted to the left in this condition)(**26**).

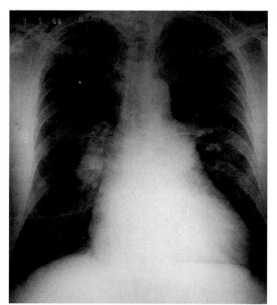

27

27 The chance association of rheumatic mitral stenosis with atrial septal defect is termed the Lutenbacher syndrome. The development of mitral stenosis will tend to accentuate the size of the left to right shunt; the chest radiograph will show cardiomegaly, left atrial enlargement and pulmonary plethora.

Primum atrial septal defect

Primum atrial septal defects are much less common than those of the secundum septum, representing about a quarter of the number of cases. In contrast to the secundum atrial septal defect, the defect occurs in the primum part of the atrial septum which is anterior to the fossa ovalis. There are often associated mitral valve abnormalities, in particular, a cleft in the anterior leaflet which may lead to mitral regurgitation. Very commonly, patients with Down's syndrome will have either a primum atrial septum defect or atrioventricular canal defects. Clinically, a primum atrial septal defect may be distinguished from a secundum defect only by the electrocardiogram, which in primum atrial septal defect will show left axis deviation together with right bundle branch block. The site of the atrial septal defect can be readily detected using cross-sectional echocardiography.

The prospects for unoperated patients with primum atrial septal defect are worse than those with a secundum defect, and include the early development of heart failure and pulmonary vascular disease.

28

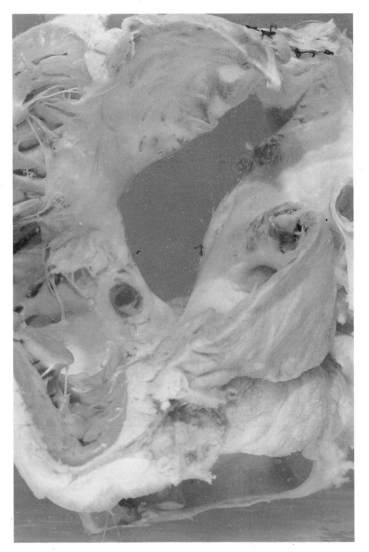

28 Macroscopic sections in primum atrial septal defect. A large defect involving the endocardial cushion can be seen together with the bridging of the mitral valve.

29, 30   In a patient with Down's syndrome it is important to search for congenital heart anomalies, particularly primum atrial septal defect and atrioventricular canal defect. Patients with Down's syndrome can be easily recognized from their facial appearance (**29**) and from the presence of a single transverse crease in the hand (**30**).

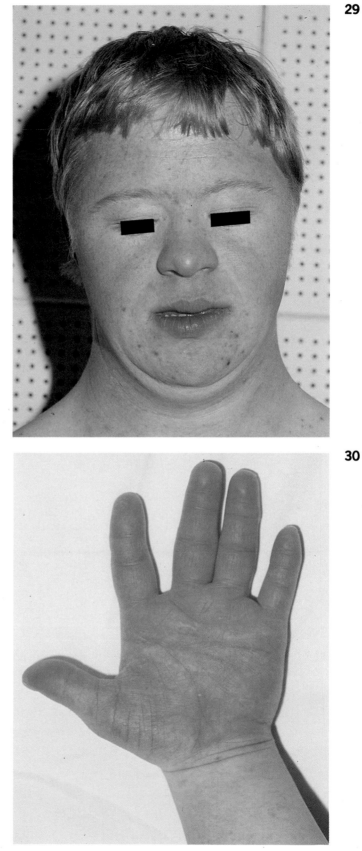

29

30

31

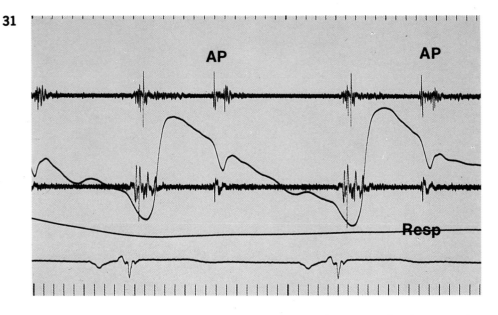

31 The auscultatory features of primum atrial septal defect include fixed splitting of the second heart sound. The cleft mitral valve may lead to the development of mitral regurgitation.

32

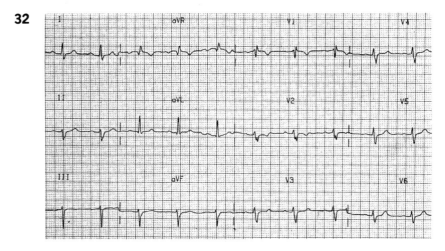

32 Characteristically, the electrocardiogram shows right bundle branch block with left axis deviation. The development of atrial fibrillation and atrial flutter is an important complication.

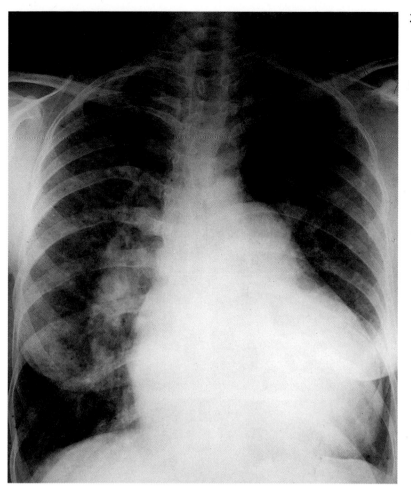

33 The chest radiograph in primum atrial septal defect cannot be distinguished from secundum atrial septal defect; the heart is enlarged, there are dilated pulmonary arteries and pulmonary plethora.

34, 35 Cross-sectional echocardiogram (parasternal short axis view). A primum defect (arrowed) can be seen (**34**; right) in the upper part of the inter-atrial septum and following surgical closure the patch (arrowed) can be seen (**34**; left). The cleft (arrowed) in the mitral valve can be shown in the short axis view (**35**; right); in the long axis view (**35**; left) the valve appears thick and redundant.

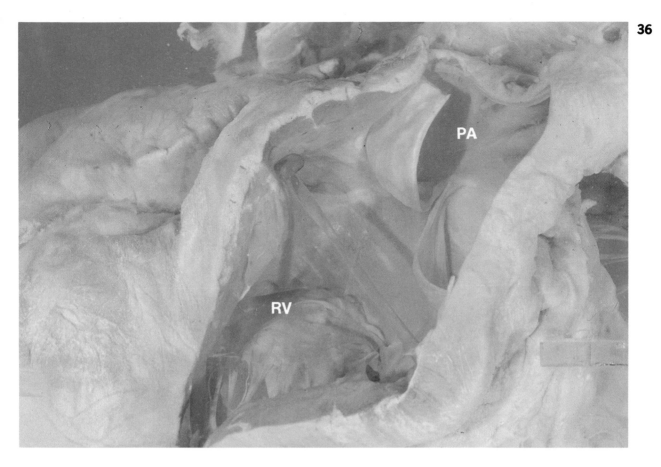

36, 37 The large left to right shunt in primum atrial septal defect leads to pulmonary artery dilatation. Pathologically this can be seen when the pulmonary artery is opened (**36**); using cross-sectional echocardiography, the gross dilatation of the pulmonary artery may be demonstrated in life (**37**)(pulmonary valve arrowed).

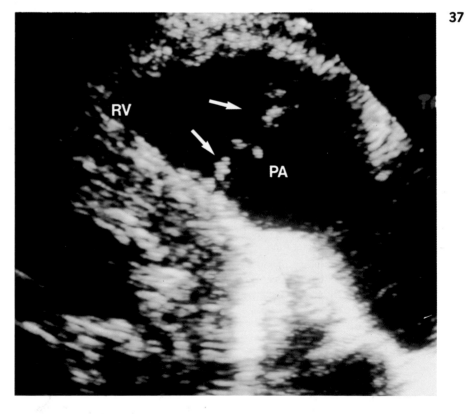

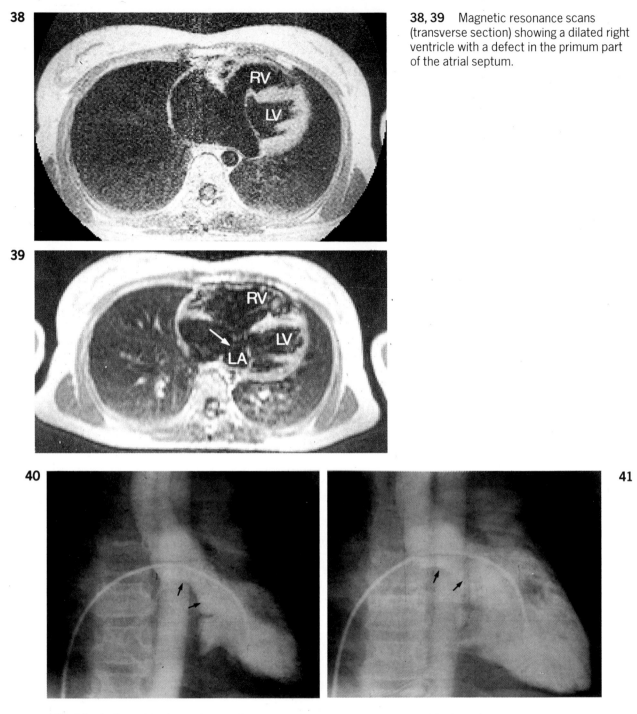

38, 39 Magnetic resonance scans (transverse section) showing a dilated right ventricle with a defect in the primum part of the atrial septum.

40, 41 Left ventricular angiogram (antero-posterior projection; systole **40**, diastole **41**) showing the typical goose-neck appearance (arrowed) associated with a primum atrial septal defect. The goose-neck is caused by elongation of the left ventricular outflow tract due to the mitral valve abnormality.

Atrioventricular canal defects and common atrium

Atrioventricular canal defects and common atrium are considered, morphologically, as similar entities and represent a more extensive form of ostium primum atrial septal defect. An atrioventricular canal defect is where the defect lies directly over the common atrioventricular valve ring and is contiguous with a ventricular defect. Common atrium is when the heart is without any vestige of an atrial septum but there are two atrial appendages. The clinical features of atrioventricular canal defects, common atrium and ostium primum atrial septal defects are all similar; the physical signs can only be differentiated by the size and presence of the ventricular component. The anatomy can best be demonstrated by cross-sectional echocardiography.

These rare abnormalities are associated with the early development of pulmonary hypertension and heart failure. Patients rarely survive beyond the fourth decade without corrective surgery.

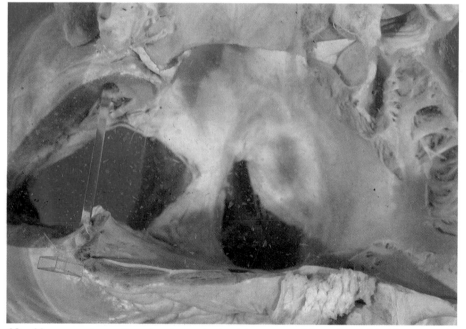

42 Macroscopic section showing a single atrium opened from the right side.

43

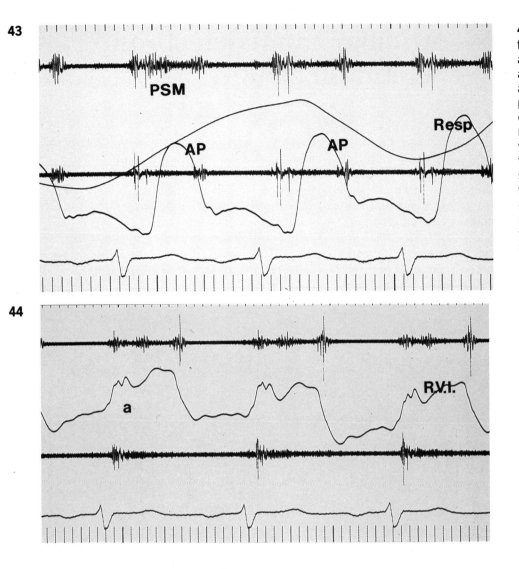

PSM

AP   AP   Resp

44

a   R.V.I.

43, 44 The clinical features of atrioventricular canal and common atrium are similar. There is a pansystolic murmur due to mitral regurgitation together with fixed splitting of the second heart sound (43). The right ventricular volume overload leads to a prominent 'a' wave in the right ventricular impulse (RVI) (44).

45 The electrocardiogram usually shows right bundle branch block with left axis deviation; there are voltage criteria for left ventricular hypertrophy. In this example there is no rSR pattern in V1.

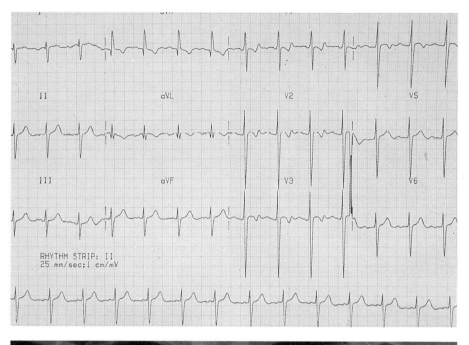

46 The chest radiograph will show evidence of pulmonary plethora with dilated pulmonary arteries. There is right ventricular predominance.

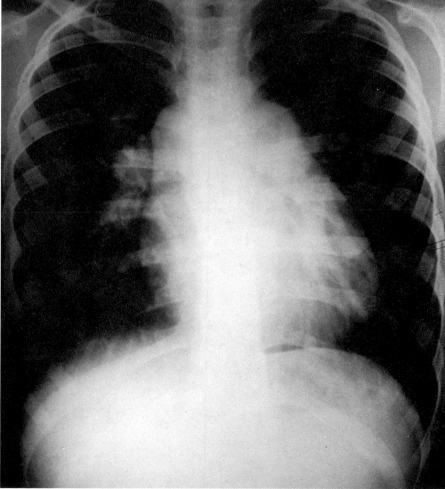

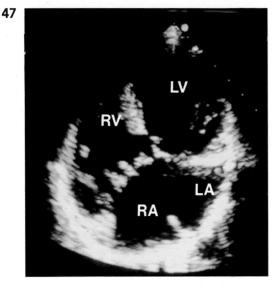

47

47—50 Figures **47** and **48** are apical four chamber views in atrioventricular septal defects. There is a ventricular septal defect, bridging of the mitral valve (arrows) and a large primum atrial septal defect with the secundum inter-atrial septum present. Both the right atrium and right ventricle are dilated. In common atrium, similar features may be observed, but in this case there is no ventricular septal defect and there is no residual inter-atrial septum (**49**). A double orifice mitral valve (arrowed) may occur, as part of the atrioventricular septal defects, and is seen in the long axis parasternal view (**50**, right) as thickening and deformation of the valve. Both orifices may be imaged directly in the short axis view (**50**, left).

48

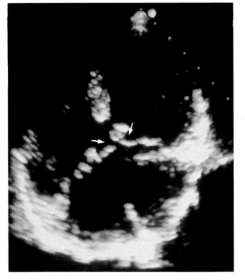

49

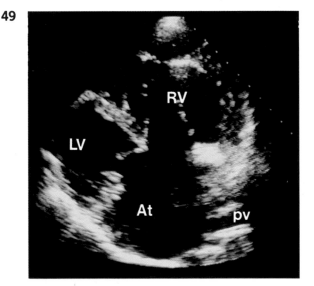

50

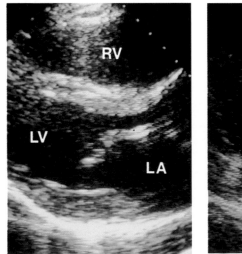
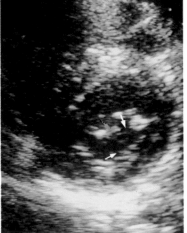

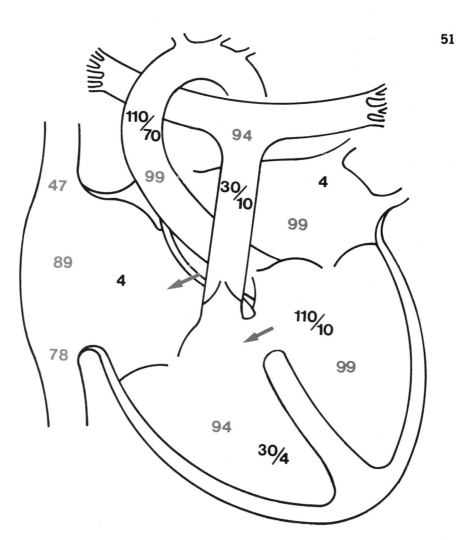

51 A saturation run in atrioventricular canal defects shows a step-up in saturation both at atrial and ventricular level, left to right, with an overall 4.8:1 shunt.

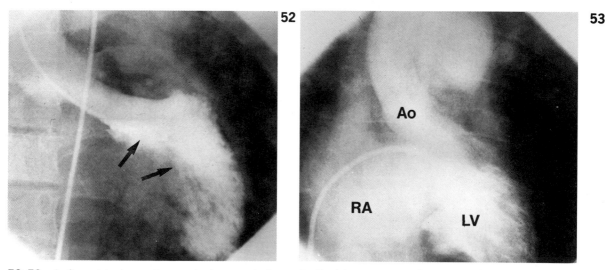

52, 53 Left ventricular angiogram (antero-posterior projection) in atrioventricular canal defect, showing filling of the atria (**52**), elongation of the left ventricular outflow tract (**53**) and an abnormal mitral valve (arrowed).

Partial and total anomalous pulmonary venous drainage

Partial anomalous pulmonary venous drainage is frequently associated with secundum atrial septal defect. Total anomalous pulmonary venous drainage occurs rarely in the adult: it often presents in neonatal life with obstruction to pulmonary venous return. Pulmonary veins may drain into the superior vena cava, right atrium, inferior vena cava or coronary sinus. Partial or total anomalous pulmonary venous drainage often cannot be distinguished clinically from secundum atrial septal defect. It may even be difficult to detect at cardiac catheterization. The natural history is similar to that of secundum atrial septal defects.

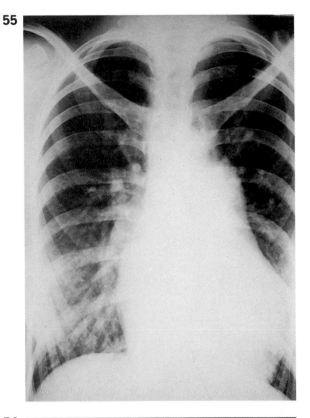

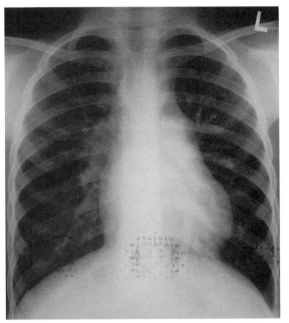

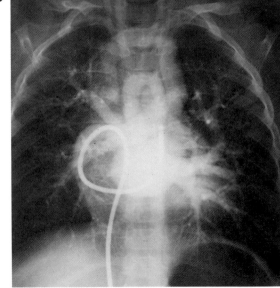

54—56 The chest radiograph in partial anomalous pulmonary venous drainage cannot be distinguished from atrial septal defect unless an anomalous vein can be identified. There will be dilated pulmonary arteries and pulmonary plethora (**54**). When the shunt is large, the heart will be enlarged and the pulmonary plethora will become more obvious (**55**). Pulmonary angiography (**56**) will demonstrate the connections of the pulmonary veins to the atria. In this example the right pulmonary veins are draining into the right atrium while the left pulmonary veins are draining into the left atrium.

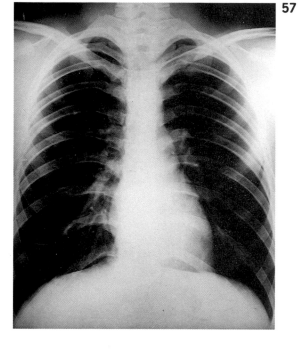

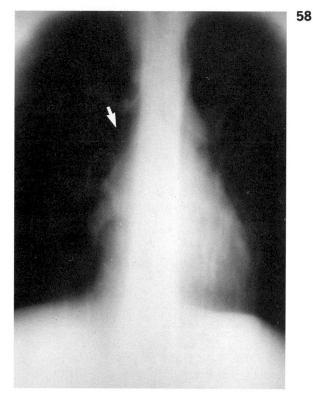

57, 58 While the anomalous vein may not be evident on the chest radiograph (**57**), tomography clearly demonstrates that the right upper pulmonary vein is draining into the superior vena cava (**58**) (arrow).

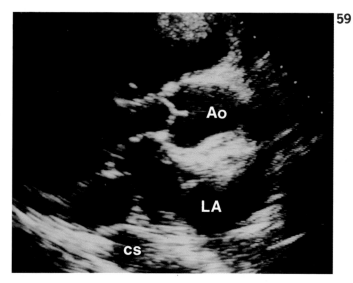

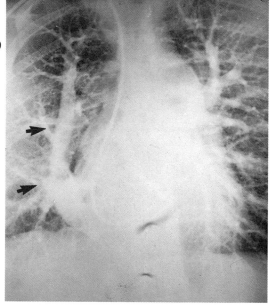

59 Cross-sectional echocardiograms (parasternal long axis view) showing a dilated coronary sinus (cs). Occasionally, as in this example, the coronary sinus is enlarged because it carries the pulmonary venous blood from the anomalous venous drainage.

60 Scimitar syndrome is a form of anomalous venous drainage in which the right upper pulmonary vein (arrowed) drains to the inferior vena cava causing an unusual but characteristic radiological appearance. The angiogram clearly delineates this vein, running downwards on the right side.

61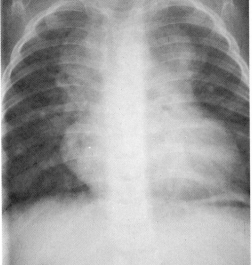

62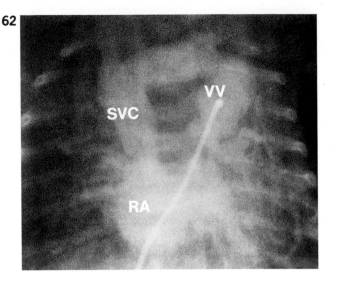

61, 62 Occasionally, total anomalous pulmonary venous drainage may be seen in the adult, but more frequently it presents in neonatal life, when there is obstruction of pulmonary venous return. This will cause the typical appearances of a 'snowman' or 'cottage loaf' when the pulmonary veins drain into the superior vena cava (**61**). This can be demonstrated by pulmonary angiography, which shows the vertical vein (VV) draining into the superior vena cava (**62**).

63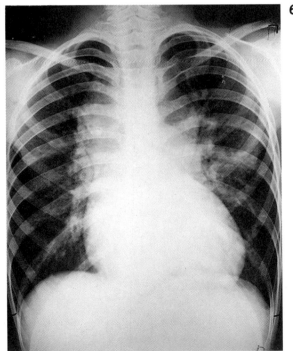

64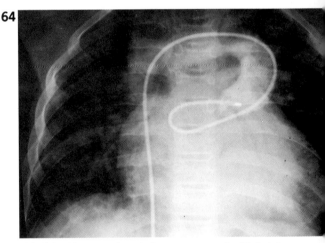

63, 64 Very rarely, adults may present with total anomalous pulmonary venous drainage, where there is evidence either of a very large shunt or the development of pulmonary hypertension. The chest radiograph will show cardiomegaly with dilatation of the upper mediastinum due to the anomalous vein (**63**). This can best be demonstrated by angiography showing the catheter passing from the superior vena cava into the pulmonary venous system (**64**). It is important to appreciate that the pulmonary venous drainage can be to sites other than the superior vena cava, including the right atrium, inferior vena cava and coronary sinus. In such circumstances the chest radiograph will not show dilatation of the upper mediastinum.

65, 66 Anomalous systemic venous drainage may occur either as an isolated phenomenon or associated with anomalous pulmonary venous drainage. If there is associated anomalous pulmonary venous drainage, then the features of dilated pulmonary artery and pulmonary plethora will dominate the chest radiograph appearances (**65**). The site of drainage of the systemic and pulmonary veins can be demonstrated by angiography showing, in this example, the right upper vein draining into the superior vena cava and the superior vena cava draining into the left atrium; an atrial septal defect is also present (**66**).

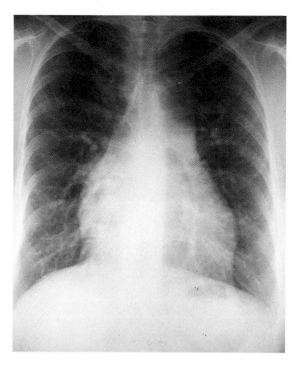

65

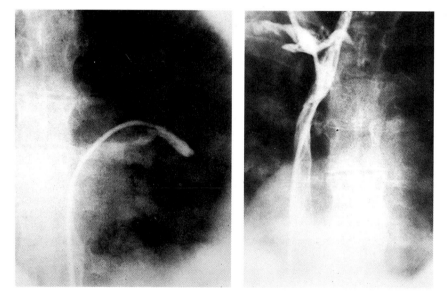

66

Ventricular septal defects

Ventricular septal defect is one of the most common forms of congenital heart disease. The defect can occur anywhere in the ventricular septum and it may be subaortic (perimembraneous), subpulmonary or beneath the tricuspid leaflet. Occasionally, ventricular septal defects may communicate between the left ventricle and right atrium (Gerbode defect); this communication may be direct or via an interventricular defect and the tricuspid valve. Ventricular septal defect may be associated with congenital pulmonary stenosis or infundibular pulmonary stenosis, or may also develop after birth as a secondary phenomenon. Prolapse of the right coronary cusp, the non-coronary cusp, or both may occur in subaortic ventricular septal defects, leading to aortic regurgitation. The characteristic clinical finding is a pansystolic murmur and the chest radiograph will show pulmonary plethora. Cross-sectional echocardiography can be used to delineate the site of the defect accurately.

Ventricular septal defects have a tendency to close spontaneously. If the defect is large, pulmonary vascular disease may occur at an early age.

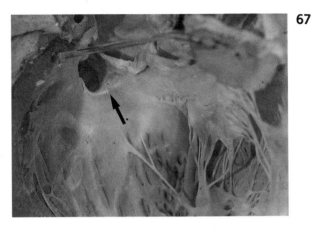

67

67   Left ventricle opened to show a subaortic ventricular septal defect (arrowed).

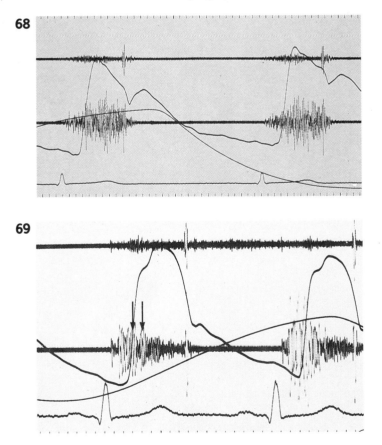

68

69

68,69   The characteristic auscultatory feature of ventricular septal defect is a pansystolic murmur at the left sternal edge engulfing the second heart sound (**68**). Where the ventricular septal defect is small, the murmur may still be very loud (Maladie de Roger). Closing muscular ventricular septal defects may have an early systolic murmur (arrows) (**69**).

70 The electrocardiogram in ventricular septal defect will be normal in small defects, but if the shunt is large will often show evidence of biventricular hypertrophy.

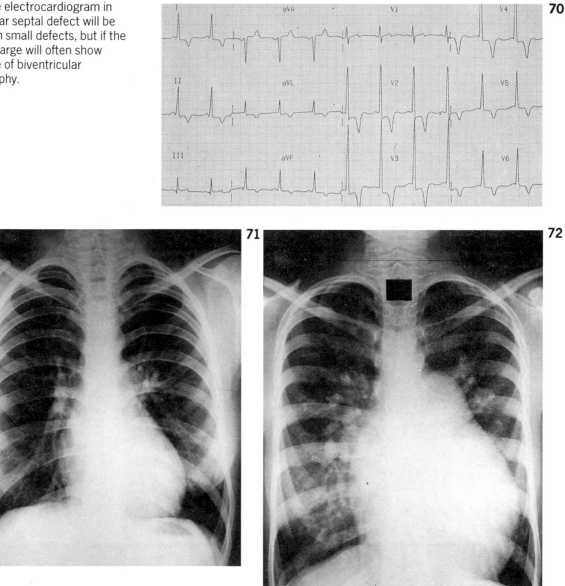

71, 72 Chest radiographs in small (**71**) and large (**72**) ventricular septal defects. The small ventricular septal defect will be associated with a normal-sized heart with slight increase in the pulmonary vascular markings. Where the ventricular septal defect is large there will be cardiomegaly with prominent pulmonary arteries and pulmonary plethora.

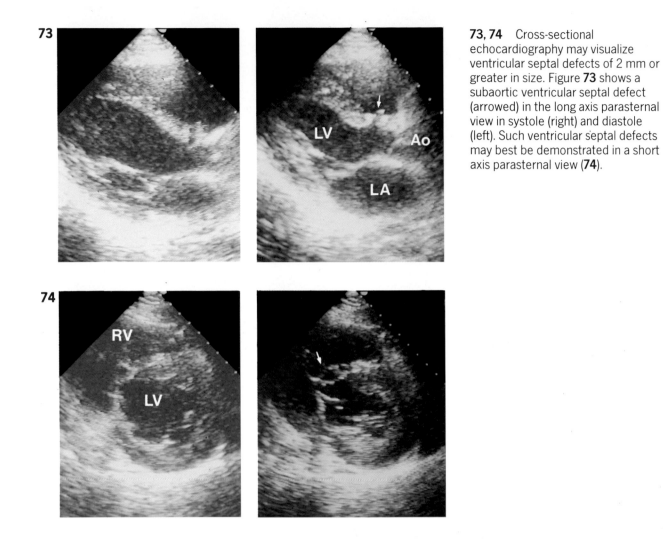

73, 74 Cross-sectional echocardiography may visualize ventricular septal defects of 2 mm or greater in size. Figure **73** shows a subaortic ventricular septal defect (arrowed) in the long axis parasternal view in systole (right) and diastole (left). Such ventricular septal defects may best be demonstrated in a short axis parasternal view (**74**).

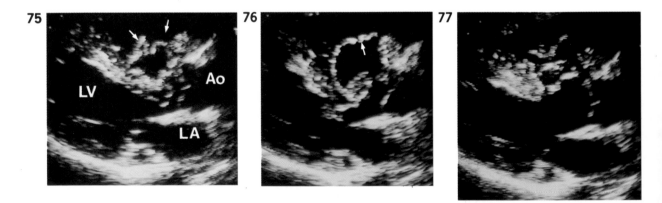

75—77 Closure of a ventricular septal defect may occur via tissue ingrowth, muscular closure or application of the tricuspid valve to the septum. The sequence of illustrations shows the movement of the tricuspid valve, when attached around the orifice of a ventricular septal defect, which lies in the left ventricular outflow tract.

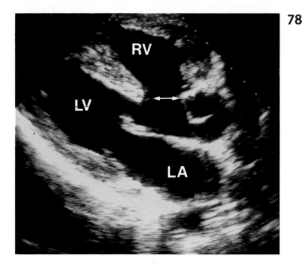

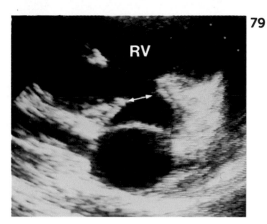

78, 79 Large ventricular septal defects may readily be demonstrated by cross-sectional echocardiography. Here a subaortic ventricular septal defect (arrowed) is seen in a parasternal view (**78**). The right ventricle is enlarged and considerable right ventricular hypertrophy can be seen. In the short axis view, the relationship of the ventricular septal defect to the right ventricular and left ventricular outflow tracts can be visualized (**79**).

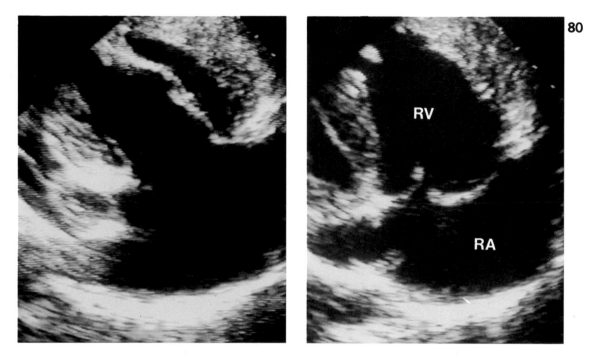

80 This figure shows dilatation of the right ventricle. Before the development of pulmonary vascular disease, the size of the right ventricle is related to the degree of left to right shunting. The right ventricle is best imaged in a parasternal inlet view, as here, which allows dilatation and hypertrophy of this ventricle to be seen (systole right and diastole left).

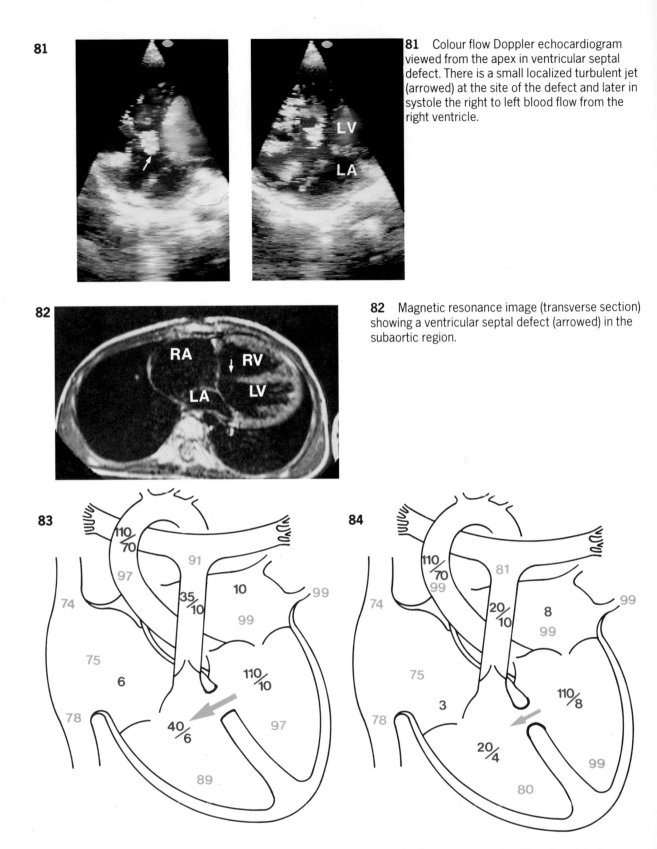

81 Colour flow Doppler echocardiogram viewed from the apex in ventricular septal defect. There is a small localized turbulent jet (arrowed) at the site of the defect and later in systole the right to left blood flow from the right ventricle.

82 Magnetic resonance image (transverse section) showing a ventricular septal defect (arrowed) in the subaortic region.

83, 84 The size of the ventricular septal defect may be estimated by the step-up in saturation at ventricular level. A small defect shows a 1.3:1 shunt; a large ventricular septal defect shows a 4:1 shunt and may be associated with some elevation of the pulmonary artery pressure.

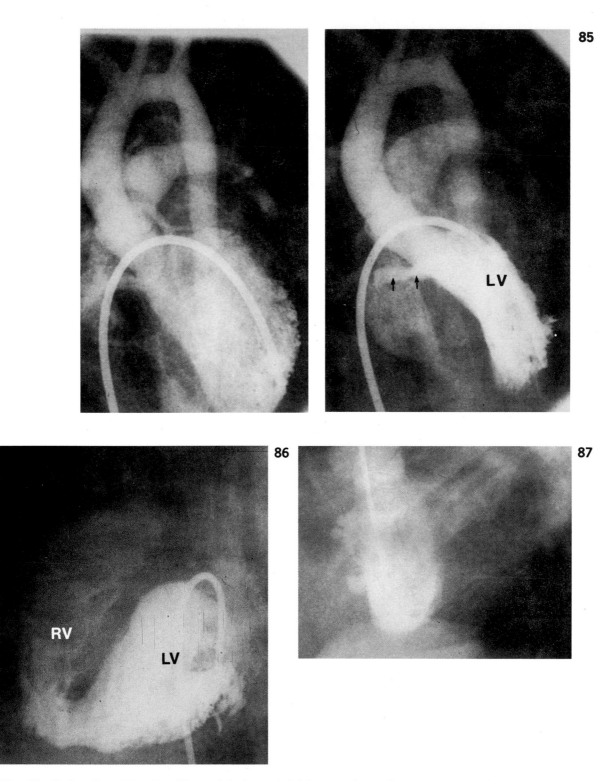

85—87   Delineation of the site of the ventricular septal defect may be made using contrast left ventricular angiography (left anterior oblique projections). The ventricular septal defect (contrast jet arrowed) may be sited in the subaortic region (**85**) or the lower part of the muscular septum (**86**). Evidence of closure of the ventricular septal defect may also be seen with the tricuspid valve (arrowed) adhering to the ventricular septum (**87**).

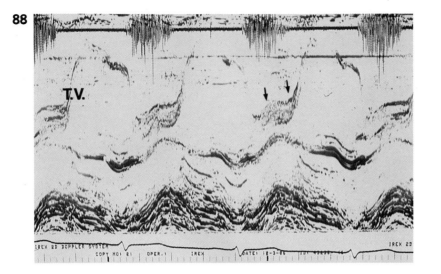

88 Ventricular septal defects may communicate between the left ventricle and right atrium (Gerbode defect). The auscultatory features will be the same as an interventricular defect. However, because of the angle of the jet from the left ventricle through to the right atrium, there will be flutter on the tricuspid valve (arrowed) which will be evident on the M-mode echocardiogram.

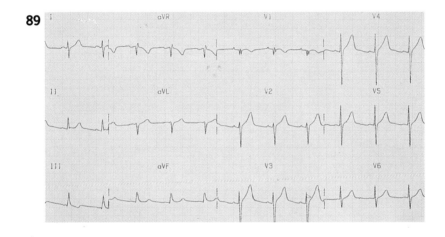

89 The electrocardiogram in Gerbode ventricular septal defect will often be normal, because the size of the shunt is usually not large.

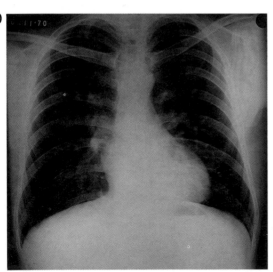

90 Chest radiograph will show a normal cardiothoracic ratio with little pulmonary plethora because, again, the shunt is not large. Right atrial enlargement may be evident.

91 Cross-sectional echocardiogram (parasternal short axis view). This shows a ventricular septal defect (arrow) which enters both the right atrium and right ventricle (arrow) either side of the tricuspid valve.

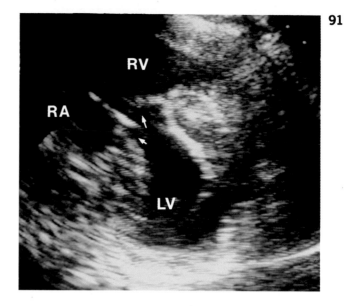

91

92, 93 Magnetic resonance scans (transverse sections) in a Gerbode defect showing the exact pathological defect (arrowed) with an interventricular defect (**92**) and then communication from the left ventricle, through the tricuspid valve into the right atrium (**93**). The net effect of this will be a direct communication between the left ventricle and right atrium.

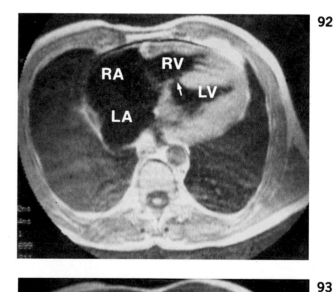

92

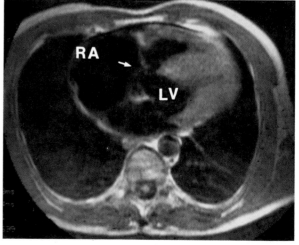

93

94

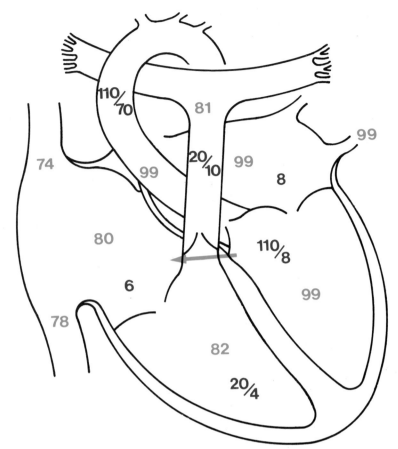

110/70
81
74
99
20/10
99
99
8
80
110/8
6
99
78
82
20/4

94 A step-up in saturations will be noticed at right atrial level and the Gerbode defect must be distinguished from an atrial septal defect by echocardiography, magnetic resonance scanning or ventriculography. The shunt is 1.3:1, left to right.

95

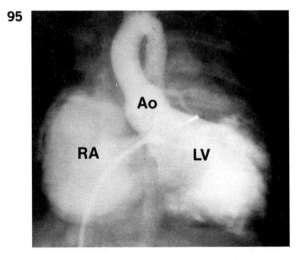

Ao
RA
LV

95 Left ventricular angiogram showing direct filling of the right atrium from the left ventricle.

96 Subaortic ventricular septal defects may be associated with prolapse of the right coronary and/or non-coronary cusps, causing aortic regurgitation. Left ventricle opened to demonstrate a subaortic ventricular septal defect with aortic valve prolapse.

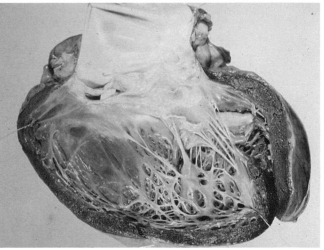

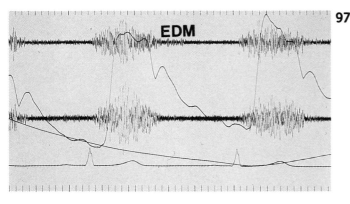

97 The characteristic auscultatory features are those of ventricular septal defect together with aortic regurgitation, causing a pansystolic murmur and an early diastolic murmur, which resembles a continuous murmur.

98 The electrocardiogram in ventricular septal defect with aortic regurgitation will show left ventricular hypertrophy and there is usually also right ventricular hypertrophy.

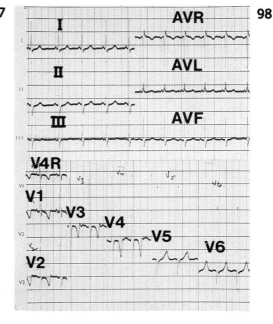

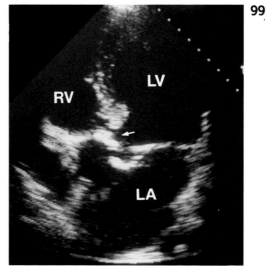

99 Cross-sectional echocardiogram (apical long axis view) showing a small subaortic ventricular septal defect (arrowed) with prolapse of the aortic valve, which results in aortic regurgitation.

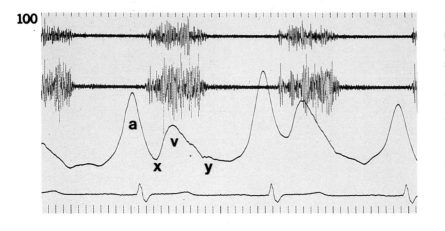

100 Ventricular septal defect may be associated with a congenital pulmonary valve stenosis. Alternatively, infundibular pulmonary stenosis may develop after birth as a secondary phenomenon. The clinical features will depend on which is the dominant lesion, but careful examination can often distinguish the presence of both lesions. If the pulmonary valve or infundibular stenosis is significant then there will be a dominant 'a' wave in the venous pressure.

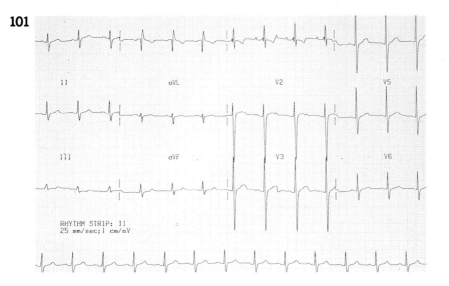

101 Electrocardiogram showing combined right and left ventricular hypertrophy which is often present in ventricular septal defect with pulmonary stenosis.

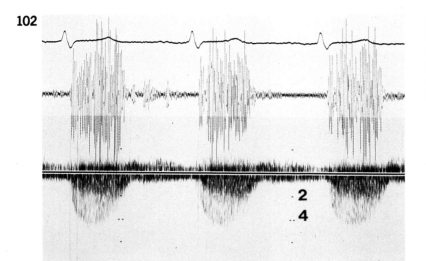

102 Doppler echocardiogram (continuous wave) of the pulmonary valve showing a large pulmonary gradient (in excess of 60 mm Hg) coincident with the murmur illustrated by phonocardiography.

103   If pulmonary stenosis is severe, in the presence of ventricular septal defect, then the right and left ventricular pressures will equalize. This may result in bidirectional shunting, which may be difficult to distinguish clinically from Fallot's tetralogy.

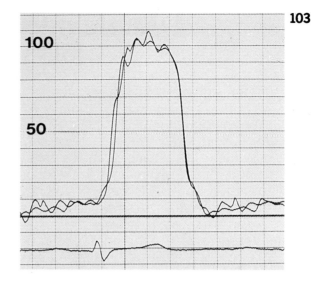

103

104,105   Left ventricular angiogram (**104**; left anterior oblique projection) showing a large subaortic ventricular septal defect with filling of the right ventricle. The right ventricular angiogram (**105**) shows severe infundibular and pulmonary valve stenosis (arrowed).

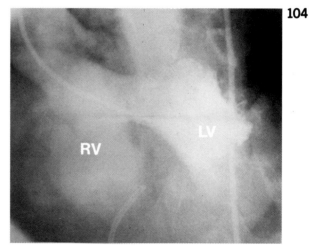

104

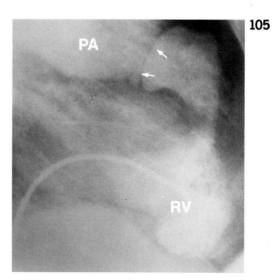

105

Double inlet left ventricle (single ventricle)

Double inlet left ventricle (single ventricle) represents a diverse group of cardiac malformations. The condition is usually characterized by both atrioventricular valves or a common atrioventricular valve opening into the same ventricle, and almost invariably there will be associated lesions, such as transposition of the great arteries, pulmonary stenosis, coarctation of the aorta or an atrial septal defect. The morphology of the ventricle is usually left, but may be right ventricular or indeterminate.

Clinical features are similar to those of a large ventricular septal defect, but may be dominated by the associated congenital lesions.

The outcome of patients with this rare condition depends largely on the associated congenital lesions. In patients with isolated double inlet left ventricle, pulmonary vascular disease will usually occur at an early age. The natural history is similar to that of a large ventricular septal defect.

106

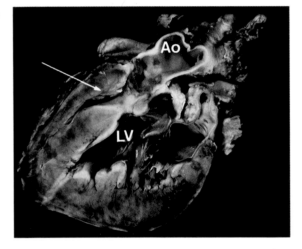

106 Macroscopic section of a double inlet left ventricle showing a rudimentary right ventricle (arrowed) lying anteriorly, communicating with a large left ventricle. Almost invariably there will be associated lesions such as transposition of the great arteries, pulmonary stenosis, coarctation or atrial septal defect. In this example, the right ventricle communicates with an anteriorly placed aorta.

107

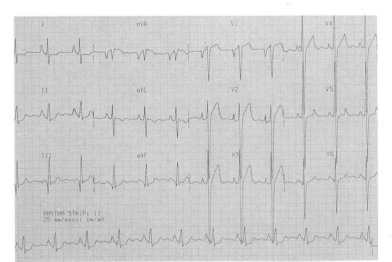

107 The electrocardiogram is non-specific (as shown).

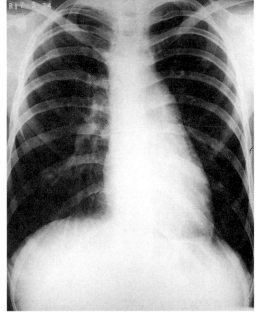

108

108 Chest radiograph will resemble a ventricular septal defect but will depend on the associated congenital lesions. In this example, the heart is not enlarged and there is a prominent pulmonary artery, but no evidence of pulmonary plethora because there is associated pulmonary stenosis. This patient had had a right Blaloch-Taussig shunt performed.

109

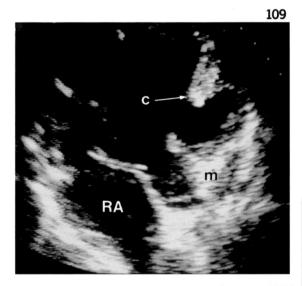

109, 110 Cross-sectional echocardiography is probably the most useful technique for delineating the morphology of the ventricle. In this example, there is a single ventricular cavity with an atretic mitral valve and a rudimentary chamber. Figure **109** (apical long axis view) shows the atretic mitral valve (m) and a crest of muscle (c) in the ventricle. The long axis parasternal view (**110**) shows the muscular rudimentary chamber (RC).

110

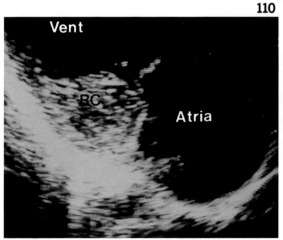

111

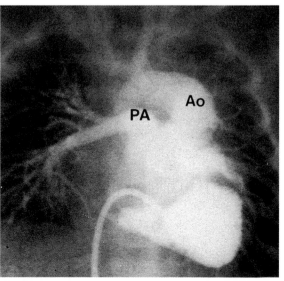

111 Left ventricular angiogram showing filling of a large ventricular cavity with both the pulmonary artery and the aorta opacifying from this cavity.

Patent ductus arteriosus

Patent ductus arteriosus is a persistent comm-unication, from foetal life, between the left pulmonary artery and the descending aorta. It is a common congenital lesion, particularly in premature infants, but in this group will often tend to close spontaneously. When present in the adult it accounts for about 5—10 per cent of all forms of congenital heart disease and is often associated with other congenital malfor-mations. The classical physical sign is that of a continuous murmur heard maximally in the upper left chest; the arterial pulse is full. The chest radiograph will show pulmonary plethora and cannot easily be distinguished from other forms of left to right shunt.

Ligation of a patent ductus arteriosus is usually recommended in all patients. When the shunt is small the major risk is infective endocarditis; with large shunts, heart failure and pulmonary hypertension may occur.

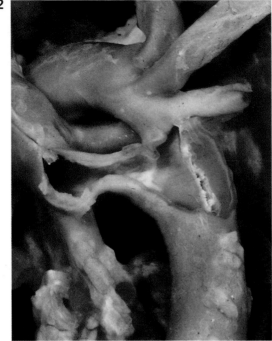

112 Aorta opened to show a patent ductus arteriosus communicating with the pulmonary artery.

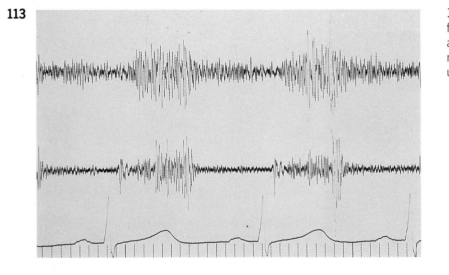

113 The classical auscultatory feature of patent ductus arteriosus is a continuous murmur heard maximally at the upper left chest.

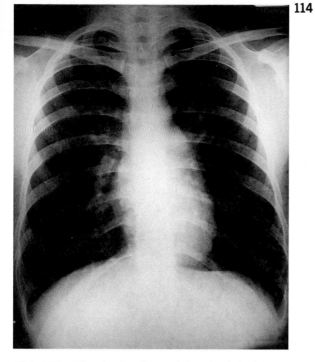

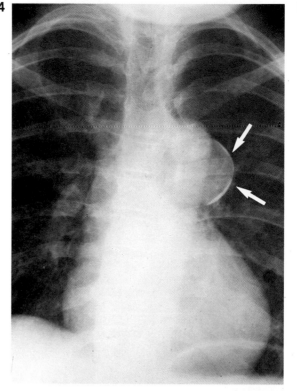

114, 115 The chest radiograph in patent ductus arteriosus will show a prominent pulmonary artery and pulmonary plethora; the heart may or may not be enlarged (**114**). With advancing years, the patent ductus arteriosus will become calcified (arrows) and the classical duct sign will be evident on the chest radiograph (**115**).

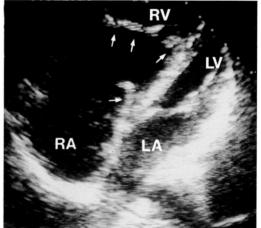

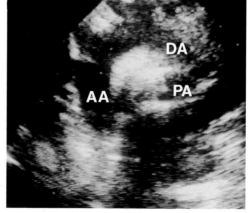

116—119 Cross-sectional echocardiography (apical four chamber view) shows that in patent ductus arteriosus the left ventricle is relatively small and there is dilatation due to volume overload of the right atrium and ventricle (**116**). In young patients it is possible to demonstrate the duct directly, by suprasternal scanning. In this example, the aortic arch is outlined with the head vessels (**117**). The duct can be seen communicating between the ascending aorta and left pulmonary artery (**117**). This may also be seen in the parasternal short axis view (**118**). Doppler ultrasound may be used to demonstrate diastolic flow within the pulmonary artery, due to the aorto-pulmonary shunt (**119**).

118

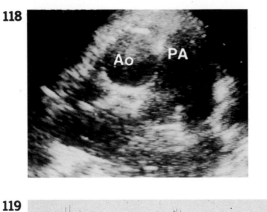

119

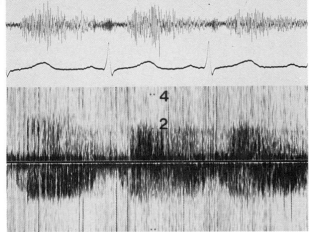

120 During catheterization the catheter will usually be passed via the left pulmonary artery into the descending aorta.

120

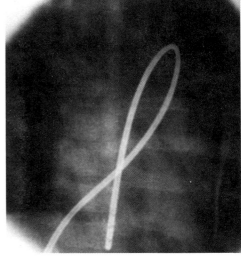

121 A saturation run in a patient with a patent ductus arteriosus will show a step-up in saturation at pulmonary artery level with a shunt of 3.1:1.

121

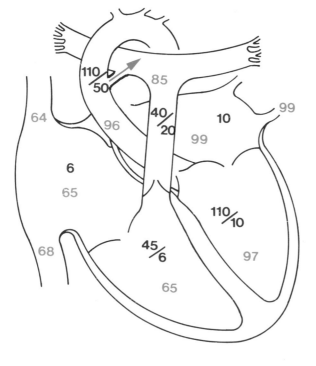

Truncus arteriosus

Truncus arteriosus is a rare condition accounting for less than 1 per cent of all congenital cardiac lesions. It may conveniently be divided into three forms. Each form has a single trunk arising from the ventricles and the three forms are divided according to the origin of the pulmonary arteries. The most common variety is where the main pulmonary artery arises from the ascending aorta and gives off the right and left pulmonary artery (type 1). Other forms include the right and left pulmonary arteries, arising from separate origins from the ascending aorta, the exact type depending on their position (type 2, type 3). Finally, type 4 truncus arteriosus is considered by some to be pulmonary atresia or an extreme form of Fallot's tetralogy, in which the pulmonary arteries arise from the descending aorta. The physical signs consist of a single second sound with systolic and early diastolic murmurs due to truncal regurgitation; the pulse will be collapsing. The diagnosis is usually confirmed on echocardiography and angiography.

Heart failure is an early complication and pulmonary hypertension develops later. Patients rarely survive beyond the third decade if this lesion is not surgically corrected.

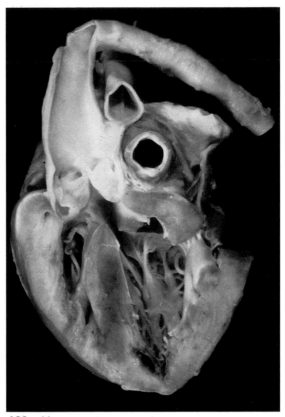

122 Macroscopic section showing a single arterial trunk arising from both ventricles, above a large ventricular septal defect (type 1 truncus).

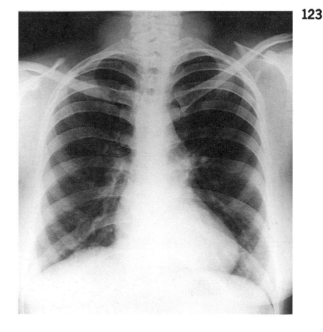

123 The chest radiograph is usually non-specific with cardiac enlargement involving both ventricles, though in this case the right is particularly involved. There is usually pulmonary plethora and the pulmonary artery is small. The left pulmonary artery has a higher than normal take off and is often at the level of the aortic knuckle.

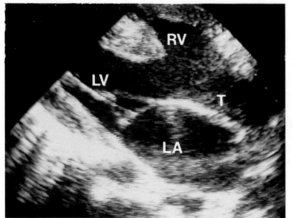

124, 125 Cross-sectional echocardiogram in truncus arteriosus. This shows a dilated and hypertrophied left ventricle with a single arterial trunk (T) arising from both right and left ventricles (**124**). The truncal valve overrides the interventricular septum. In diastole (**125**) there is prolapse of the truncal valve (arrows) resulting in truncal regurgitation. This occurs because the valve is four cuspid and readily becomes regurgitant with dilatation of the arterial root.

125

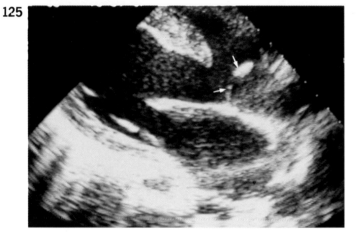

126

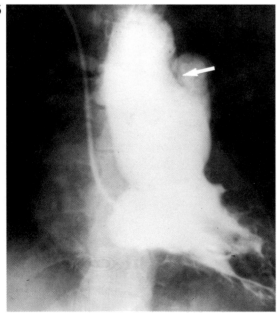

126—128 Left ventricular angiogram (anteroposterior projection **126**; lateral projection **127**) showing filling of the aorta and pulmonary artery (arrow) from the common trunk (type 1 truncus). Figure **128** shows an aortogram in a patient with a type 2 truncus with the separate pulmonary arteries (arrowed) arising from the aorta.

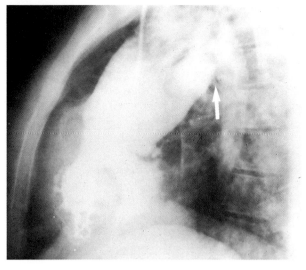

127

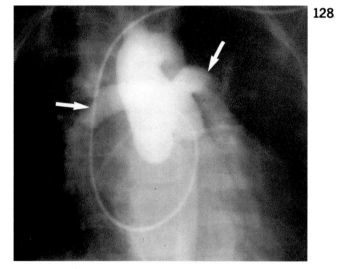

128

129 Although there are four types of truncus, there are in fact a number of variations, as shown in this aortogram where the left pulmonary artery arises from the ascending aorta while the right pulmonary artery arises from the descending aorta (hemitruncus).

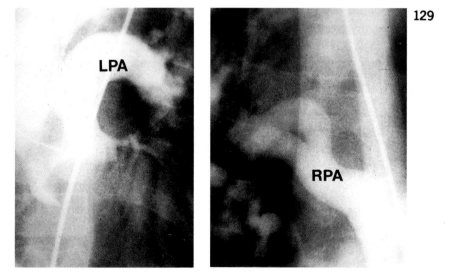

129

LPA

RPA

Eisenmenger syndrome

Eisenmenger syndrome was originally described as pulmonary hypertension occurring secondary to a ventricular septal defect. The term has now been broadened to include pulmonary hypertension occurring secondary to any form of left to right shunt. The Eisenmenger syndrome is an important irreversible complication of left to right shunts; with the increase in early detection and correction of these conditions at an early age, this syndrome is becoming progressively less common. Patients with the Eisenmenger syndrome will be cyanosed. Irrespective of the underlying cause, the classical physical findings are those of right ventricular hypertrophy and a loud pulmonary component to the second heart sound. The cross-sectional echocardiogram can delineate the underlying aetiology of the Eisenmenger syndrome, but cardiac catheterization or Doppler echocardiography are necessary to determine the pulmonary artery pressure.

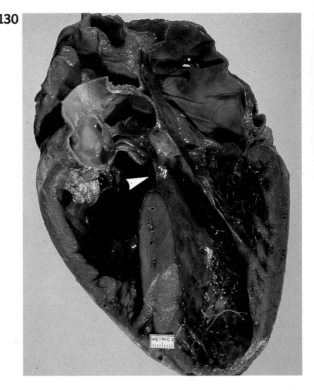

130 Long axis section showing dilated left and right ventricles with a subaortic ventricular septal defect (arrow).

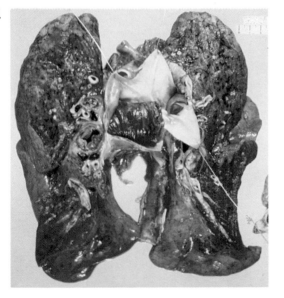

131 Excised lungs and open pulmonary arteries in Eisenmenger syndrome. At the end stages of this condition, thrombosis (arrow) of the main pulmonary artery occurs.

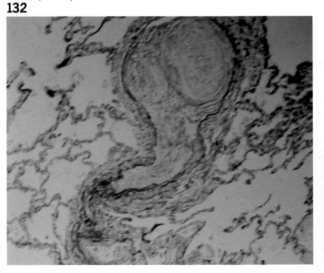

132 Histological section of the lungs in Eisenmenger syndrome will show evidence of pulmonary hypertensive changes with intimal proliferation, recannulization and dilated sinusoids.

133—135 Patients with Eisenmenger syndrome will be cyanosed, best appreciated around the lips and tongue (**133**). There will also be finger clubbing (**134**) and clubbing of the toes (**135**). Classically, these patients will also be polycythaemic which contributes to the peripheral cyanosis.

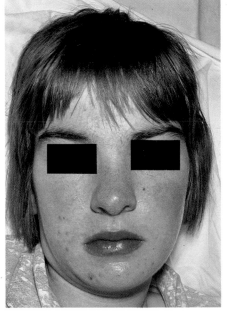

133

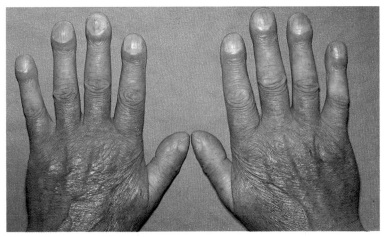

134

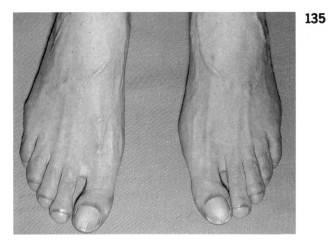

135

136

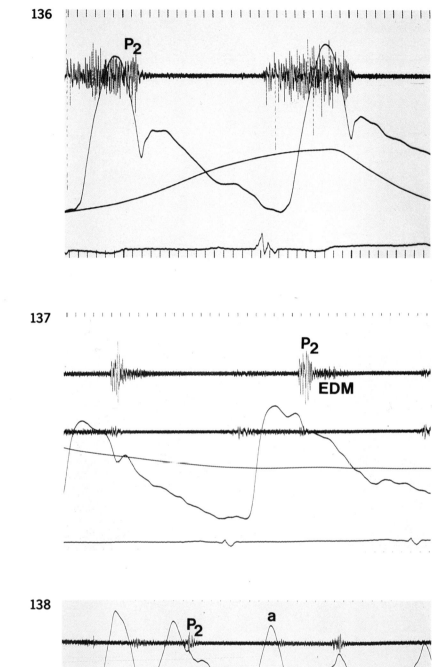

P₂

137

P₂

EDM

138

P₂

a

x

v

y

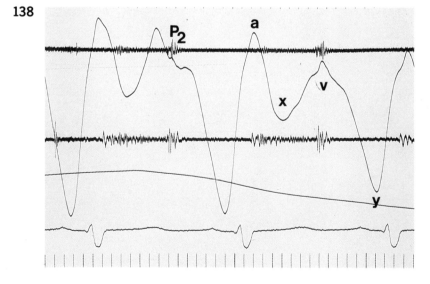

136—139 The auscultatory features of Eisenmenger syndrome will include evidence of pulmonary hypertension, irrespective of the cause; a loud pulmonary component of the second heart sound will be evident. Figure **136** shows an Eisenmenger ventricular septal defect in which the pulmonary component of the second heart sound is loud and in addition there is a pansystolic murmur arising from the ventricular septal defect; however, occasionally there may be no murmur at all. Similarly, in patent ductus arteriosus with pulmonary hypertension, the features will be dominated by a loud pulmonary closure sound and often there is an early diastolic murmur of secondary pulmonary regurgitation (**137**). Clinical examination of the venous pressure will show a dominant 'a' wave in the presence of an elevated jugular venous pressure (**138**) and the right ventricular impulse will be accentuated with a prominent 'a' wave (**139**).

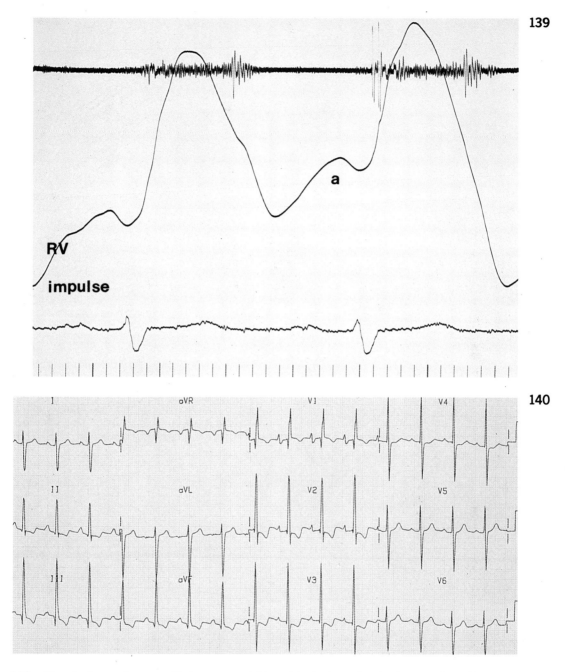

140 The electrocardiogram will show gross right ventricular hypertrophy, irrespective of the underlying cause.

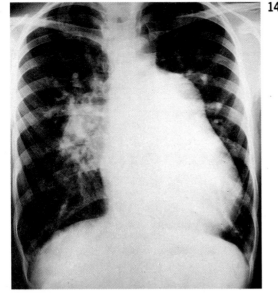

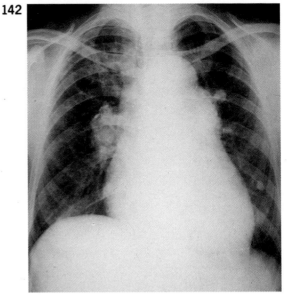

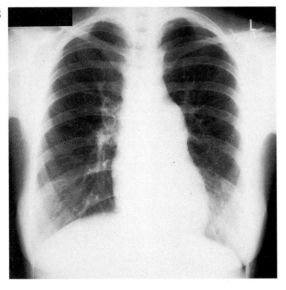

141—144 Chest radiograph will be dominated by the presence of a prominent pulmonary artery and, classically, pruning of the peripheral pulmonary arteries (**141**). Often, there is cardiomegaly (**142**), but occasionally the heart size may be normal (**143**). Evidence of the underlying aetiology may be found on the chest radiograph. Calcification of the pulmonary arteries (arrows) may occur in all causes of Eisenmenger syndrome (**144**).

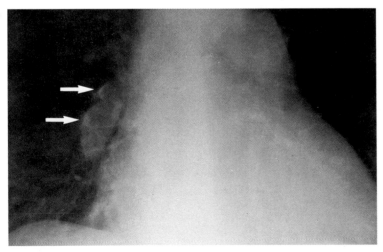

145—148 The cross-sectional echocardiogram can delineate the underlying aetiology of Eisenmenger syndrome. Figure **145** is an apical four chamber view showing a large subaortic ventricular septal defect. The right ventricle is enlarged and there is hypertrophy of the septum. Note that the inter-atrial septum bows from right to left, reflecting the increase in right atrial pressure above left atrial pressure. Figure **146** shows a short axis view in the same patient, allowing for a further appreciation of the size of the ventricular septal defect and the extent of right ventricular hypertrophy in Eisenmenger syndrome. Parasternal long axis view (**147**; systole left, diastole right) showing dilatation of the right ventricle with a small left ventricle in an Eisenmenger ventricular septal defect. There is also a pacemaker within the right ventricle. Continuous wave Doppler (**148**) can be used to determine right ventricular pressure. The peak velocity of tricuspid regurgitation may be measured by continuous wave Doppler from the parasternal window and this velocity is directly related to pulmonary artery pressure. In this patient with Eisenmenger syndrome, the right ventricular systolic pressure and therefore pulmonary artery systolic pressure equals approximately 60 mm Hg.

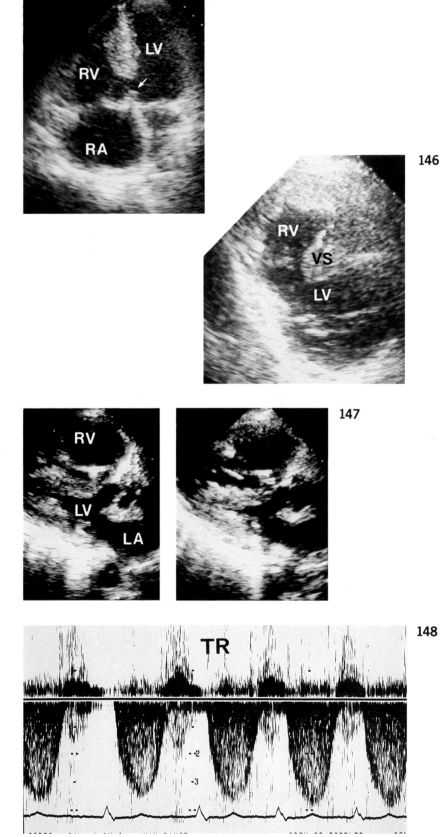

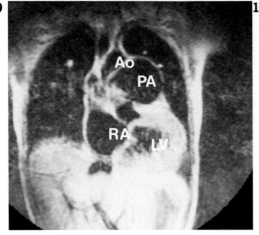

149

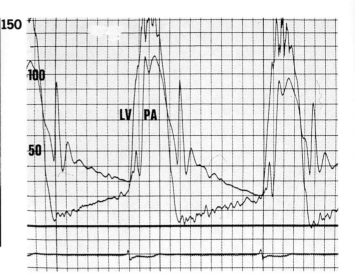

150

149 Magnetic resonance scans can be used to delineate the anatomy, as in this example of Eisenmenger patent ductus arteriosus.

150 Elevation of the pulmonary artery pressure to systemic levels is a characteristic feature of Eisenmenger syndrome.

151

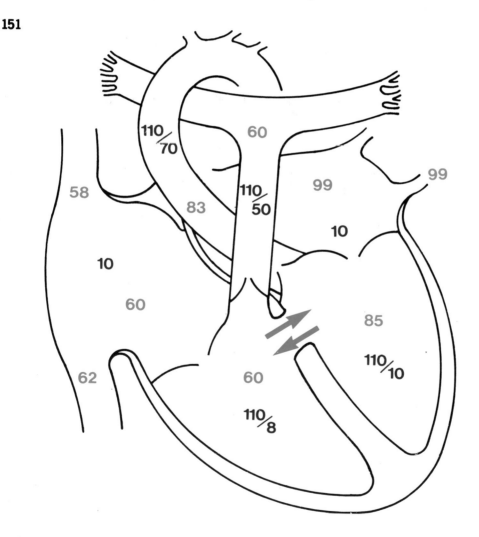

151 Saturation run will show evidence of a bidirectional shunt with desaturation evident in the left ventricle and aorta, in an Eisenmenger ventricular septal defect.

Pulmonary stenosis

Pulmonary stenosis may occur at valve level, subvalve or above the valve in the branch pulmonary arteries. Subvalvular pulmonary stenosis may occur in association with a valvular pulmonary stenosis or in conjunction with other congenital lesions, such as ventricular septal defect or Fallot's tetralogy. The physical signs are those of an ejection systolic murmur and in the presence of valvular pulmonary stenosis there will be an ejection click. In severe pulmonary valve stenosis, pulmonary closure will be delayed and soft. The chest radiograph will show pulmonary artery dilatation and cross-sectional and Doppler echocardiography can be used to delineate the site of obstruction and its severity.

Pulmonary stenosis is a relatively common congenital cardiac lesion accounting for up to 10 per cent of all congenital malformations. The prognosis is good in the adult, though if pulmonary stenosis is severe, right heart failure may ensue.

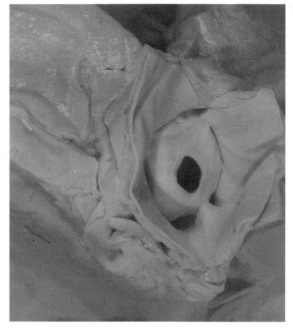

152

152 A congenitally stenosed pulmonary valve viewed from above.

153 There is a strong association between Noonan's syndrome (neck webbing, low set hair line and hypertelorism) and pulmonary stenosis.

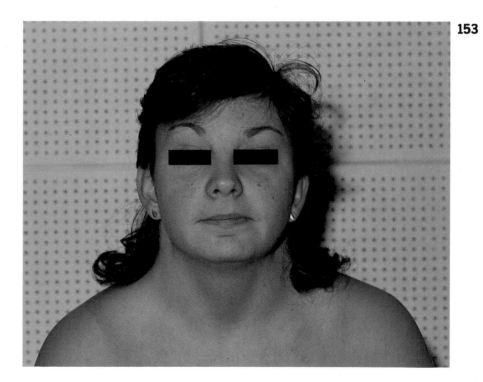

153

154

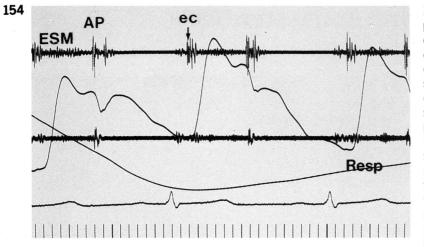

154—157 In mild congenital pulmonary stenosis there will be an ejection click (EC), normal splitting of the second heart sound and an ejection systolic murmur (**154**). In severe pulmonary stenosis the ejection click is still present, but the systolic murmur is loud and long and pulmonary closure is delayed (**155**). Following pulmonary valvotomy the systolic murmur will be quieter, but evidence of pulmonary regurgitation frequently present (**156**). The venous pressure in pulmonary stenosis is dominated by a predominant 'a' wave due to right ventricular hypertrophy (**157**).

155

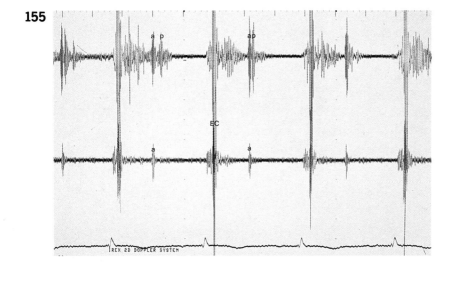

156

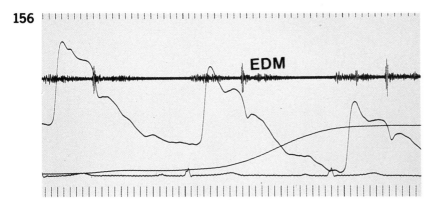

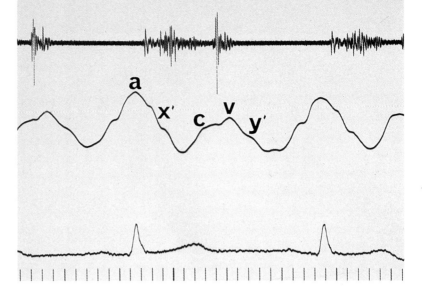

157

158,159 Electrocardiogram in mild pulmonary stenosis may be normal or show evidence of right atrial hypertrophy (tall P waves) (**158**). With more severe pulmonary stenosis there will be evidence of right ventricular hypertrophy (**159**).

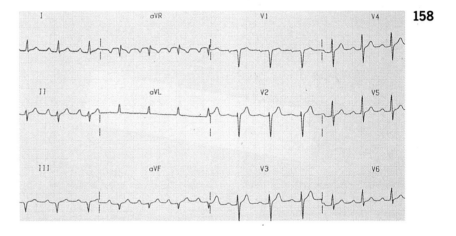

158

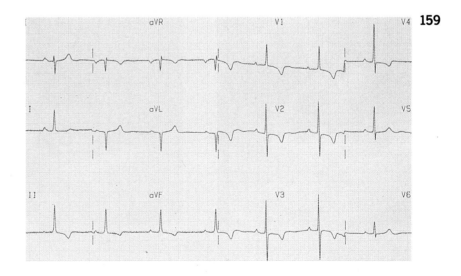

159

160

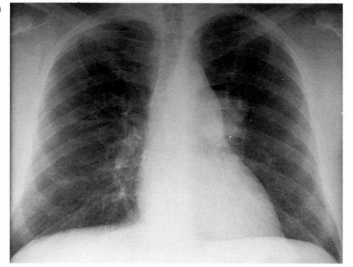

160 The classical feature on the chest radiograph is pulmonary artery dilatation.

161

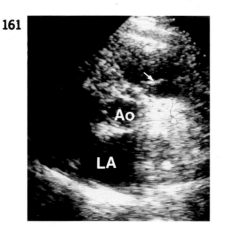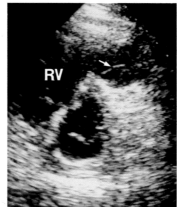

161—163 Cross-sectional echocardiograms in pulmonary stenosis. The parasternal short axis view shows the pulmonary valve (arrow) to be thick and have impaired movement (**161**, systole left, diastole right). Figure **162** shows more marked thickening of the pulmonary valve (arrow) with calcification. In severe long standing pulmonary stenosis (**163**) there will be dilatation and impairment of function of the right ventricle, as seen on this right ventricular inlet view.

162   **163**

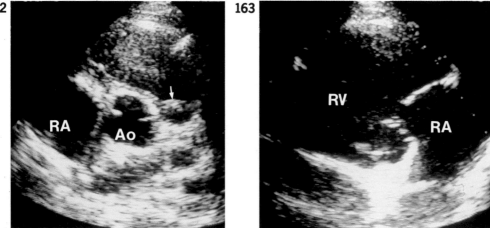

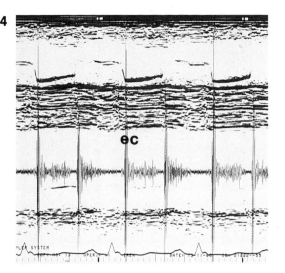

165
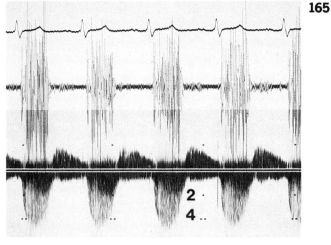

164—166 Figure **164** shows the mechanism of the ejection click (ec) in pulmonary stenosis. The top trace shows the M-mode echocardiogram of the pulmonary valve. The timing of the rapid checking of the thickened valve is coincident with the ejection click, seen on the phonocardiogram below. The Doppler echocardiogram may allow assessment of the severity of pulmonary stenosis. Continuous wave Doppler, in this example, shows a gradient of more than 4 m/s across the pulmonary valve (**165**); this represents a pulmonary valve gradient in excess of 60 mm Hg. Following pulmonary valvotomy, pulmonary regurgitation may be demonstrated by Doppler echocardiography; pulmonary regurgitation (PR) is seen as high frequency signals towards the transducer and there is no residual pulmonary stenosis (**166**).

166
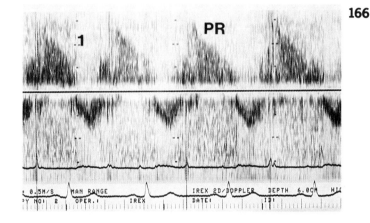

167
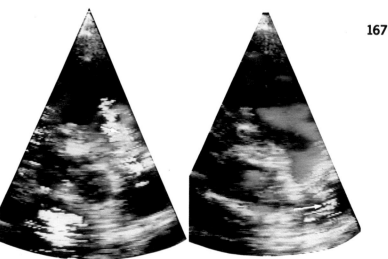

167 Colour flow Doppler (parasternal short axis view) showing a localized eccentric turbulent jet of pulmonary stenosis across a dysplastic valve (arrow right) and pulmonary regurgitations (arrow left).

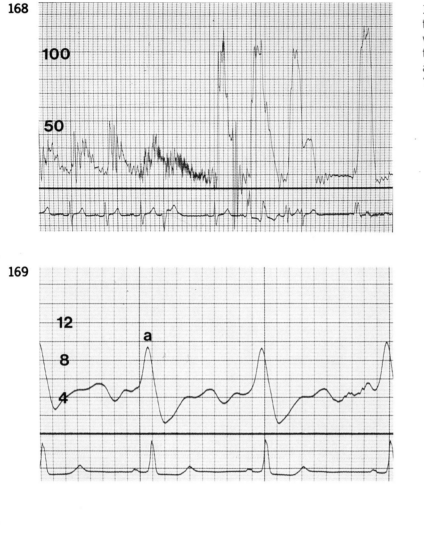

168,169 Withdrawal tracing from the pulmonary artery to the right ventricle will show a gradient across the pulmonary valve (**168**). The right atrial pressure trace will show a tall 'a' wave (**169**).

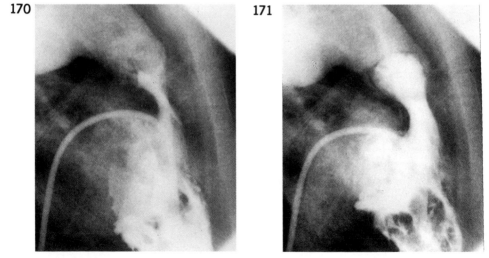

170,171 Right ventricular angiograms (lateral projection; systole **170**, diastole **171**) showing a domed, thickened pulmonary valve with infundibular shut down during systole.

172,173 Figure **172** shows the balloon across the pulmonary valve and in the left hand image the narrowing can be seen indenting the balloon. Following successful dilatation the balloon becomes fully inflated (right hand image). Figure **173** shows the angiogram before and after dilatation.

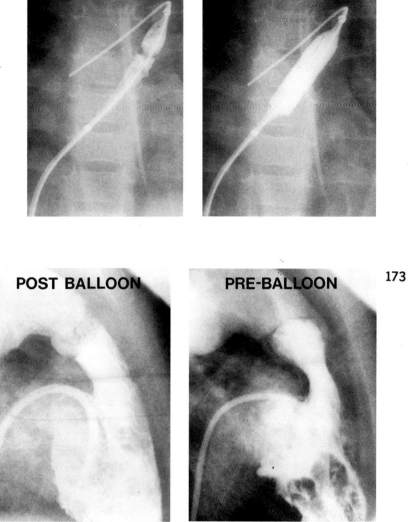

174 Branch pulmonary stenosis may be isolated, but usually it occurs in association with valvular pulmonary stenosis or Fallot's tetralogy. The physical signs are of an ejection systolic murmur which is maximal over the area of stenosis. Pulmonary arteriography will demonstrate the lesions (arrows).

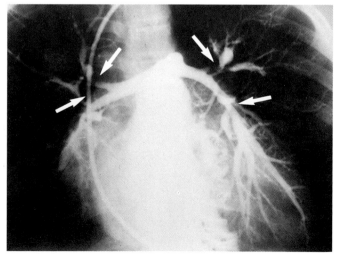

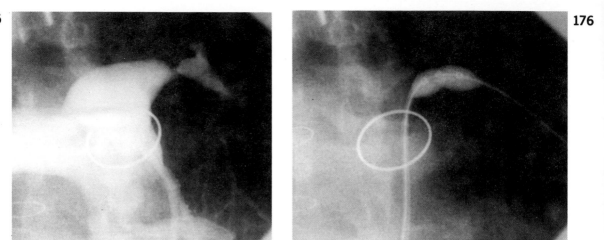

175,176 Branch pulmonary stenosis at the site of previous surgery (**175**) can also be dilated using balloon angioplasty. Figure **176** shows indentation of the balloon catheter by the branch stenosis.

177

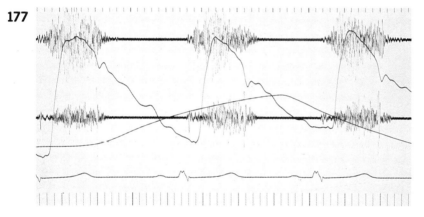

177 Subvalve or infundibular pulmonary stenosis may occur either as an isolated phenomenon or in association with ventricular septal defect, Fallot's tetralogy or valvular pulmonary stenosis. The auscultatory features are similar to valvular pulmonary stenosis, but there will be no ejection click. Figure **177** shows an ejection systolic murmur, delayed pulmonary component of the second heart sound and no ejection click.

178

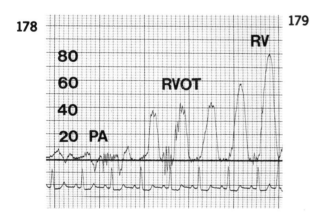

178 Haemodynamic tracing showing withdrawal from pulmonary artery to right ventricle in which two gradients can be seen, the first at valve level and again at infundibular level.

179

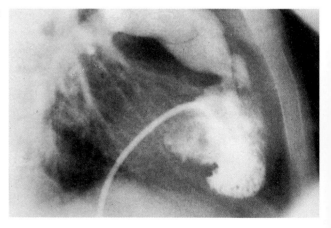

179 Right ventricular angiogram (lateral projection) showing severe infundibular stenosis with thickening of the pulmonary valve.

Fallot's tetralogy

Fallot's tetralogy is one of the commonest forms of cyanotic congenital heart disease seen in the adult. It consists of pulmonary stenosis, a subaortic ventricular septal defect with aortic override and right ventricular hypertrophy. The physical signs are dominated by the presence of pulmonary stenosis and ventricular septal defect in a patient who is cyanosed. Cardiac morphology may be demonstrated by cross-sectional echocardiography and angiography.

The natural history is variable and is determined principally by the severity of right ventricular outflow tract obstruction. Twenty-five per cent of untreated patients with Fallot's tetralogy will die in the first year of life. A few survive into the fourth and fifth decades untreated. Total correction is now performed in all patients in whom this diagnosis is made; however, it does not prevent the development of serious ventricular arrhythmias in adult life.

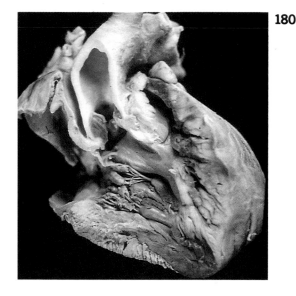

180

180 Right anterior oblique equivalent long axis echo cut of the heart to show overriding aorta, pulmonary stenosis, ventricular septal defect and right ventricular hypertrophy.

181,182 Patients with Fallot's tetralogy are classically cyanosed and have finger clubbing (**181**). When extreme, the fingers may appear like drumsticks (**182**).

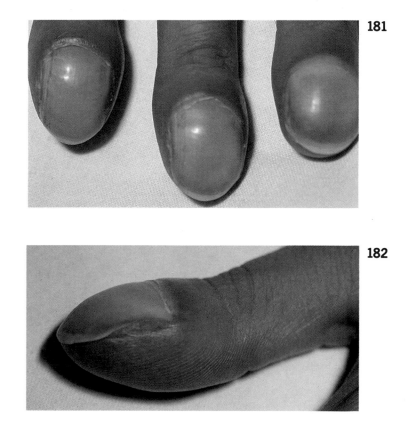

181

182

183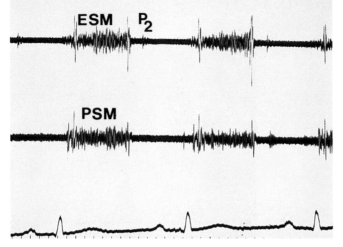

184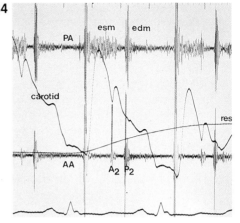

183,184 The auscultatory features of Fallot's tetralogy include a pansystolic murmur, due to the ventricular septal defect, with a soft delayed pulmonary closure, due to the pulmonary stenosis (**183**). In addition, there will also be an ejection systolic murmur in the pulmonary area, due to pulmonary stenosis. This murmur may still be evident after closure of the ventricular septal defect and repair of the pulmonary outflow tract (**184**). Following repair of Fallot's tetralogy the murmur of pulmonary regurgitation may also be present.

185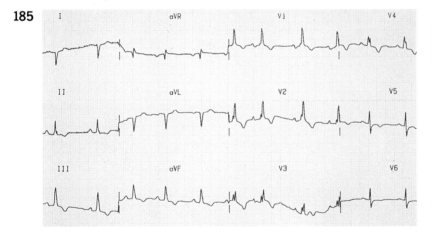

185 The electrocardiogram in Fallot's tetralogy shows evidence of right atrial and right ventricular hypertrophy.

186,187 Chest radiograph in Fallot's tetralogy classically shows a boot-shaped heart with an uptilted apex, due to right ventricular hypertrophy, small pulmonary arteries and pulmonary oligaemia (**186**). A right aortic arch occurs in 25 per cent of patients with Fallot's tetralogy or may occur as a normal variant, as in this example (**187**).

186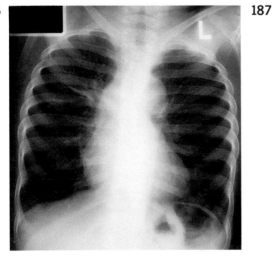

187

188 Cross-sectional echocardiogram (parasternal long axis; systole left, diastole right) in Fallot's tetralogy. This demonstrates the overriding of the aorta across the interventricular septum in the region of the subaortic ventricular septal defect. Right ventricular hypertrophy may be seen.

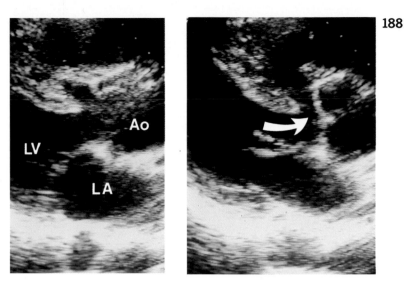

188

189 Haemodynamic investigation in patients with Fallot's tetralogy will demonstrate the presence of balanced ventricular pressures and evidence of bidirectional shunting.

189

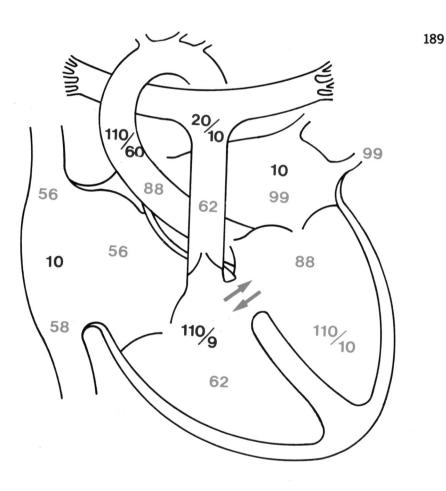

190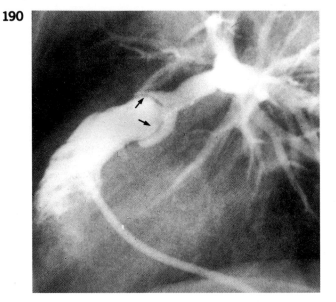

191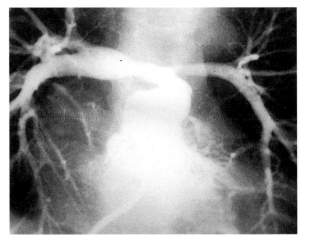

192

190—192 Right ventricular angiogram (lateral projection) showing pulmonary valve stenosis (**190**) with a domed pulmonary valve (arrows). Frequently, the main and branch pulmonary arteries are under-developed, seen in this right ventricular angiogram (**191**; right anteroposterior cranial tilted view). Left ventricular angiography will show aortic override, filling of the right ventricle and filling of the pulmonary arteries (**192**).

Pulmonary atresia

Absence of the pulmonary valve with subsequent hypoplasia of the pulmonary arteries is termed pulmonary atresia. Patients with this condition do not live to adult life without corrective surgery in the absence of an associated ventricular septal defect. This condition is rare, causing severe cyanosis. The auscultatory features are variable and depend on the underlying associated lesions; collateral murmurs may be heard. These patients will usually require cardiac catheterization to establish the complete morphological diagnosis.

Patients with this condition usually undergo either palliative surgery or corrective surgery at an early age.

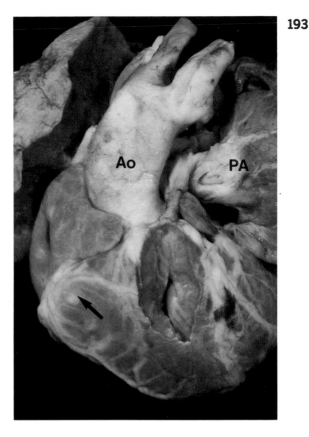

193

193 Pulmonary atresia in adult life is only seen when there is an associated ventricular septal defect. Figure **193** shows an unopened heart viewed from above, sectioned to show the blind ending right ventricle (arrow). There is a large aorta and the main pulmonary artery is not connected to the right ventricle.

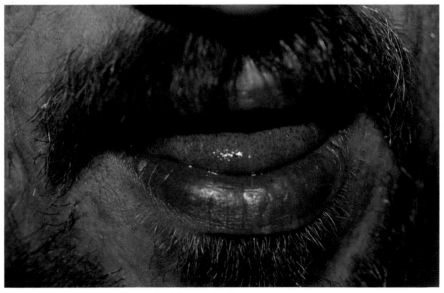

194

194 Cyanosis is present in pulmonary atresia and is usually evident around the lips and tongue.

195

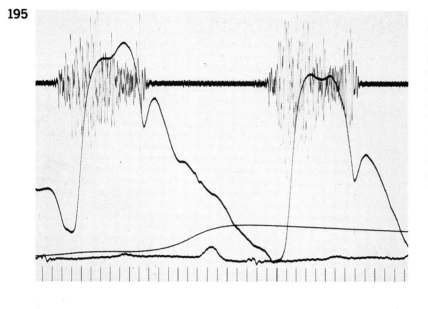

195—197 The auscultatory features of pulmonary atresia are complicated and depend on the underlying lesions. Evidence of a ventricular septal defect is found as a loud pansystolic murmur at the left sternal edge (**195**). Frequently there is associated aortic regurgitation where an early diastolic murmur may be present (**196**). The pulmonary closure sound will be absent (**195, 196**). The presence of collaterals will be detected by continuous murmurs heard over the back (**197**).

196

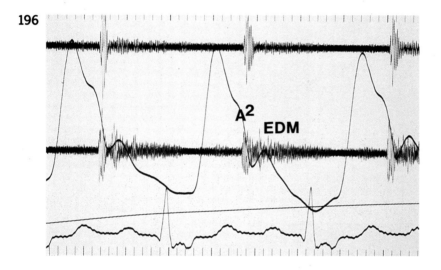

A^2 EDM

197

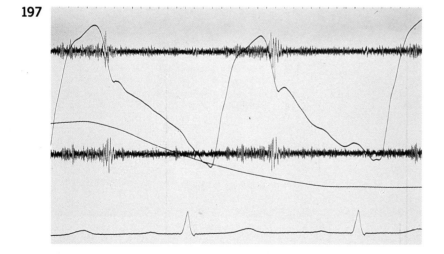

198 Electrocardiogram of a patient with pulmonary atresia and a ventricular septal defect, will show right ventricular hypertrophy.

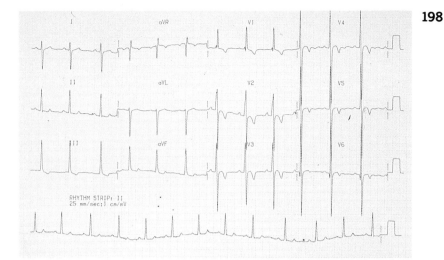

199 Chest radiograph in pulmonary atresia will show small pulmonary arteries with mild cardiomegaly. A right arch is frequently present and often the collaterals can be seen, shown here in the right upper lobe.

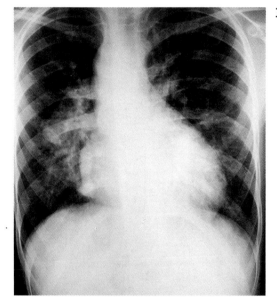

200 Cross-sectional echocardiogram in pulmonary atresia can be used, in adults, to demonstrate the absence of the pulmonary artery, the presence of an outflow ventricular septal defect (arrow) and an overriding aorta (left). Colour Doppler echocardiogram (left) shows a turbulent jet (orange) passing from the aorta into the right ventricle.

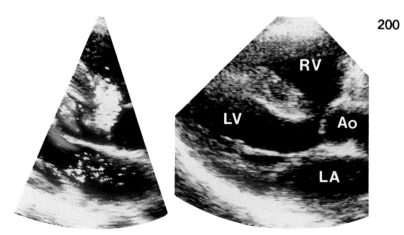

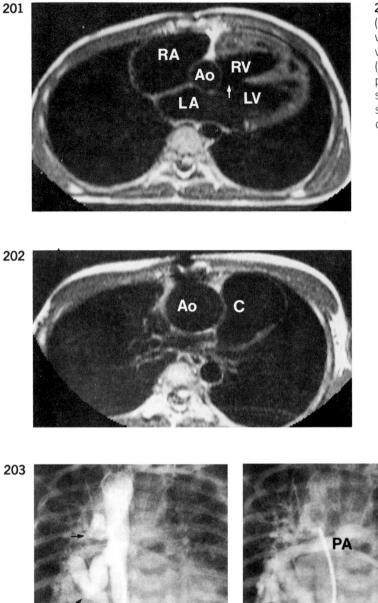

201, 202 Magnetic resonance scanning (transverse section) shows the subaortic ventricular septal defect (arrow) and right ventricular hypertrophy in pulmonary atresia (**201**). A section at the level of the carina, in a patient who had undergone a Rastelli repair, shows the aorta and conduit (c), but in addition shows small pulmonary arteries and systemic collaterals (**202**).

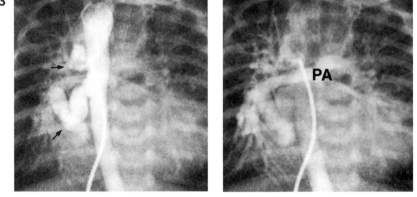

203 Descending aortogram in pulmonary atresia will demonstrate the presence of large collaterals (arrows) (left hand image); the later phase shows filling of the main pulmonary artery and the right and left pulmonary arteries (right panel).

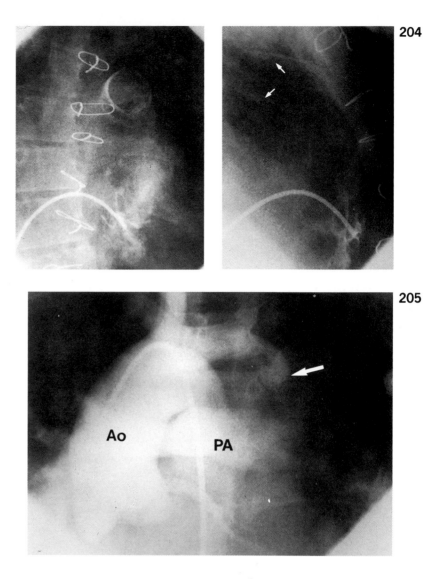

Ao PA

204—206 Most patients with pulmonary atresia will
present in adult life having undergone cardiac surgery. Total
correction is now performed using a Rastelli repair with a
conduit (arrows) from the right ventricle to the pulmonary
artery (calcified in this example) (**204**). In the past, most
patients underwent shunting procedures; the most
common was the Blalock Taussig shunt shown in this
aortogram, with filling of the pulmonary arteries via a left
Blalock Taussig shunt (arrow) (**205**). Glenn shunts were also
performed where the superior vena cava was anastomosed
to the right pulmonary artery (**206**); however, this
procedure is rarely performed nowadays since it frequently
thrombosed.

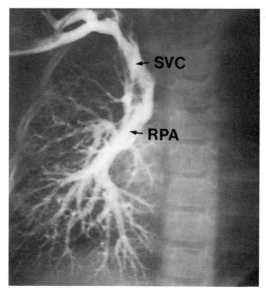

206

SVC

RPA

Ebstein's anomaly

Ebstein's anomaly is uncommon and occurs in less than 1 per cent of patients with congenital heart disease. It is characterized by a congenital defect of the tricuspid valve in which the leaflets are displaced downwards into the right ventricle. The leaflets are deformed and the anterior leaflet is invariably large and sail-like. Patients with Ebstein's anomaly are usually mildly cyanosed but occasionally this can be severe. The diagnosis of Ebstein's anomaly is best made using cross-sectional echocardiography.

There is a wide morphological spectrum of the disease and some patients may remain asymptomatic throughout their lives. In contrast, others may present in the first week of life with right heart failure and cyanosis. The electrocardiogram, in about 5 per cent of patients with Ebstein's anomaly, shows a type B Wolf-Parkinson-White syndrome and patients with Ebstein's anomaly in general are prone to the development of tachyarrhythmias.

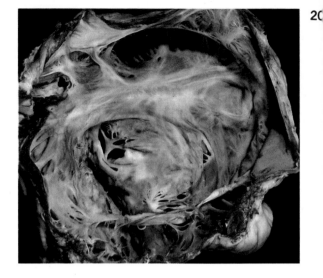

207   Right atrium opened to show the downward displacement of the tricuspid valve into the right ventricle; the valve is deformed and redundant.

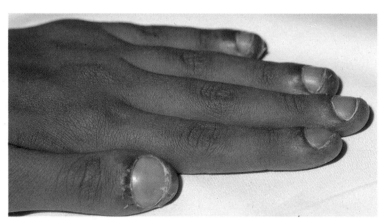

208   Some patients with Ebstein's anomaly are cyanosed due to shunting from right to left at atrial left. Occasionally. when this is extreme, finger clubbing may be present.

209 The auscultatory features of Ebstein's anomaly include a split first heart sound and a third and fourth heart sound. There may be a pansystolic murmur due to tricuspid regurgitation.

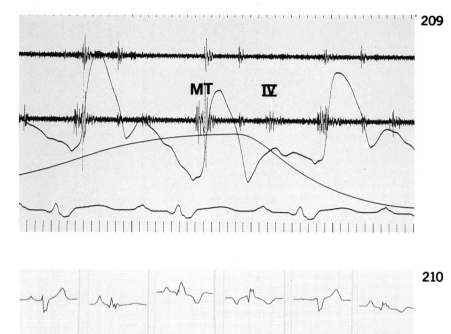

210 The electrocardiogram shows a prolonged PR interval and right bundle branch block.

I II III aVR aVL aVF

V1 V2 V3 V4 V5 V6

211 Chest radiograph in Ebstein's anomaly will show cardiomegaly and a rounded shaped heart with underfilling of the lung fields.

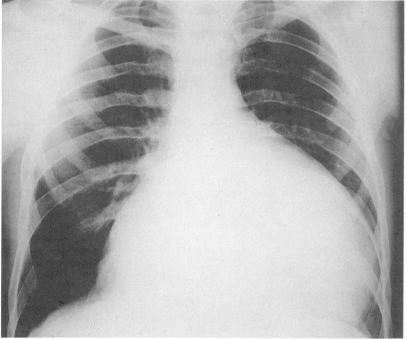

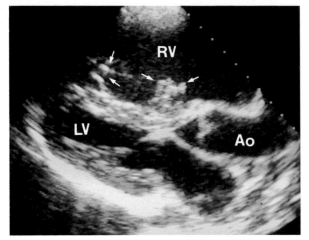

212—216 Cross-sectional echocardiography is the method of choice for imaging the abnormal tricuspid valve (arrowed) and its attachments. Figure **212** shows a parasternal long axis view in Ebstein's anomaly; the left ventricle is small and the right ventricle is dilated, redundant tricuspid valve tissue can be seen. Imaging from the apex through the cardiac cycle (**213-215**) shows that the tricuspid valve is attached not in its normal position at the level of the mitral valve, but displaced downwards along the interventricular septum. Colour flow Doppler echocardiography apical long axis view showing a turbulent multicoloured jet of tricuspid regurgitation in early (left) and late (right) systole from the downward displaced tricuspid valve (**216**).

213   214   215

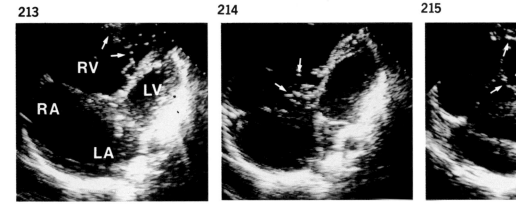

216

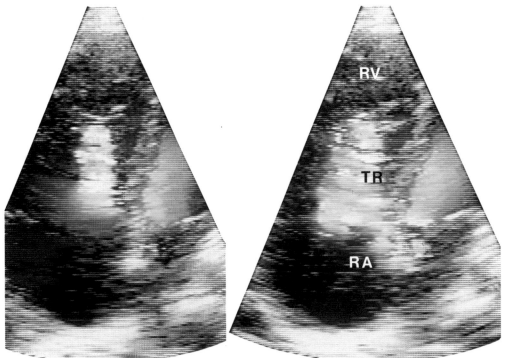

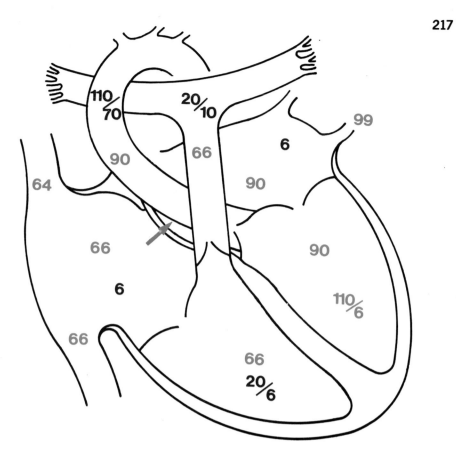

217 Haemodynamic investigation of patients with Ebstein's anomaly will show an elevated right atrial pressure and evidence of right to left shunting at atrial level.

Tricuspid atresia

Tricuspid atresia accounts for 1—3 per cent of all forms of congenital heart disease, in which the right atrium fails to open into the right ventricle through an atrioventricular valve. Characteristically, the electrocardiogram shows left axis deviation and left ventricular hypertrophy and there will be pulmonary oligaemia on the chest radiograph. Patients only survive to adult life if there is associated ventricular septal defect or patent ductus arteriosus; the severity of obstruction to pulmonary blood flow will predominantly determine the natural history. In the long term, prognosis will also be influenced by the left ventricular function.

Patients with tricuspid atresia are severely cyanosed from birth and clubbing will occur, usually after the age of 2 years. Most patients will have a loud systolic murmur due to the ventricular septal defect and a mid diastolic murmur due to augmented flow across the mitral valve. The diagnosis is made by cross-sectional echocardiography and angiography.

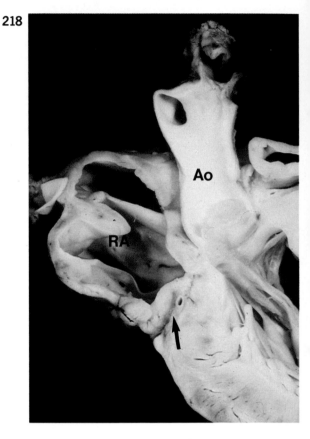

218

218 Opened heart to show a large right atrium, unperforated tricuspid valve (arrow) and a hypoplastic right ventricle.

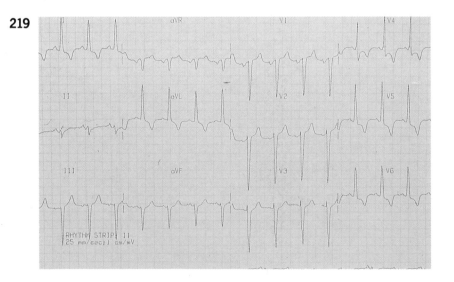

219

219 Electrocardiogram in tricuspid atresia will show left ventricular hypertrophy with left axis deviation.

220 Chest radiograph in tricuspid atresia will show pulmonary oligaemia with hypoplasia of the main pulmonary artery. Classically, not shown in this example, the right heart border is straight.

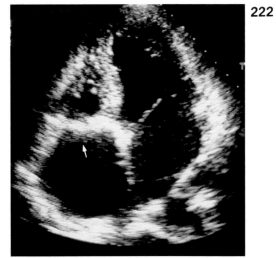

221, 222 Cross-sectional echocardiogram (apical four chamber view) in systole (**221**) and diastole (**222**) showing an atretic tricuspid valve (arrow) with a normal-sized right and left atrium. The right ventricle appears small and the ventricular septal defect is not seen in this view.

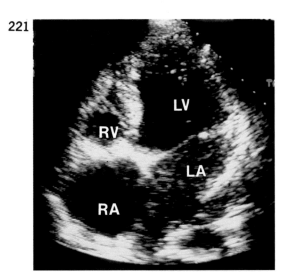

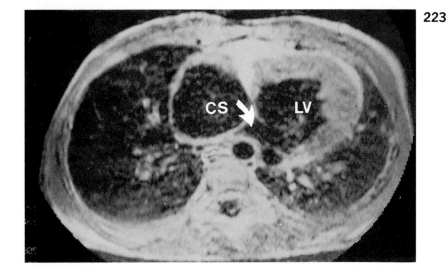

223 Magnetic resonance image (transverse section) showing absence of the right ventricle with a large hypertrophied left ventricle. In addition, the inferior vena cava and coronary sinus are dilated.

224

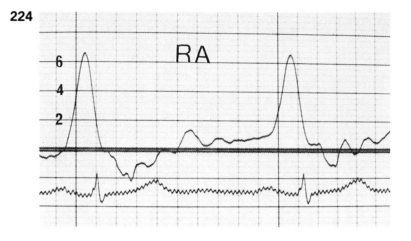

224 Haemodynamic tracing in tricuspid atresia shows a dominant 'a' wave in the right atrial pressure tracing.

225

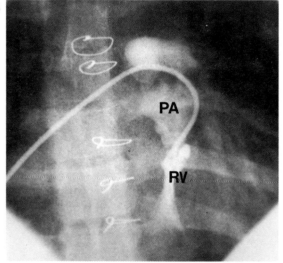

225—227 Right ventricular angiogram (antero-posterior projection) with the catheter passing via a Fontan shunt into the pulmonary artery and back into the right ventricle, showing the diminutive right ventricle which communicates with the right pulmonary artery (**225**). Classically, the angiogram features of tricuspid atresia are obtained on the right atrial angiogram (**226**) with filling of the right atrium to the left atrium and then the left ventricle; there is a triangular filling defect where the right ventricular inflow is normally seen (arrows). Following the Fontan procedure, right atrial injection will show the anastomosis, with filling of the pulmonary arteries (**227**).

226

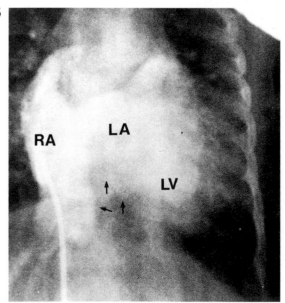

227

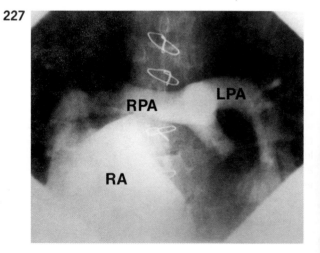

Complete transposition of the great arteries

Complete transposition of the great arteries is a common cyanotic congenital heart lesion, presenting in neonatal life, in which the aorta arises from the right ventricle and the pulmonary artery arises from the left ventricle. While accounting for up to 7 per cent of all forms of congenital heart disease, only 10 per cent of patients will survive the first year of life without surgery. In approximately half of all cases, transposition of the great arteries is an isolated condition, but such patients will not survive to adult life without corrective or palliative surgery. All patients presenting in adult life who are unoperated will have a large intracardiac shunt as an associated condition. Auscultation will reveal a single second heart sound, but the diagnosis is usually made using cross-sectional echocardiography or angiography.

Most neonates will undergo a Rashkind balloon septostomy soon after birth with radical correction (Mustard's procedure, Senning's procedure and arterial switch) before the development of irreversible pulmonary hypertension. If there is an associated ventricular septal defect a Rastelli procedure is performed, in which a conduit is placed through the ventricular septal defect from the right ventricle to the pulmonary artery.

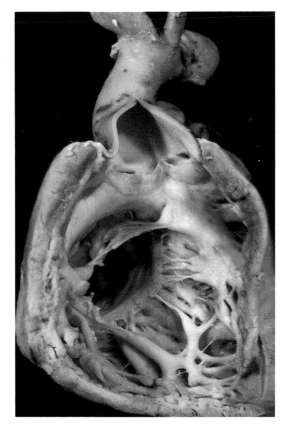

228

228, 229 Opened right ventricle showing communication between the right ventricle and aorta in transposition of the great arteries (**228**). Opened left ventricle showing communication between the left ventricle and the pulmonary artery in transposition of the great arteries (**229**).

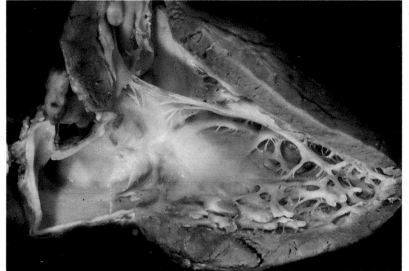

229

230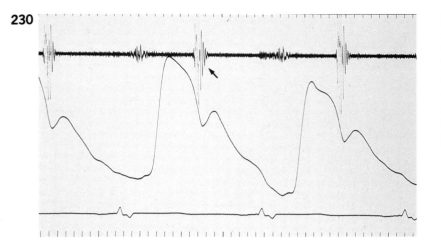

230 Auscultation in transposition of the great arteries will reveal the presence of a single loud second sound (arrow). The other auscultatory features will depend on the presence of any other underlying condition, such as a ventricular septal defect or pulmonary stenosis.

231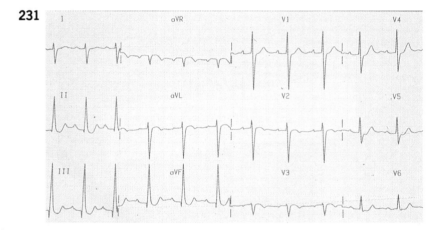

231 Electrocardiogram will show right axis deviation and there may be right ventricular hypertrophy (not shown in this example).

232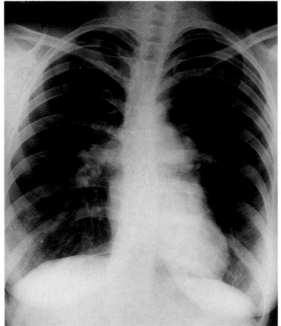

232 Chest radiograph in transposition of the great arteries will reflect, to some extent, the underlying conditions that are present in addition to the transposition of the great arteries. In this example, with transposition of the great arteries, there is a ventricular septal defect with pulmonary hypertension; the heart size is normal, the pulmonary arteries are enlarged with pulmonary plethora and there is a right aortic arch.

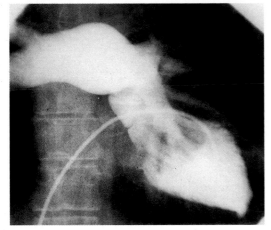
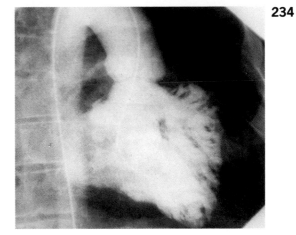

233, 234 Left ventriculogram (antero-posterior projection) showing the pulmonary artery arising from the left ventricle (**233**). Right ventriculogram (antero-posterior projection) showing the aorta arising from the right ventricle (**234**).

235
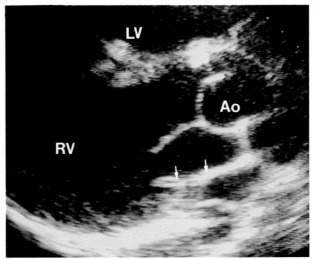

235, 236 Cross-sectional echocardiograms in transposition of the great arteries, following a Mustard procedure in which systemic and pulmonary venous return is redirected using a pericardial baffle (B,arrow) within the atria.

236
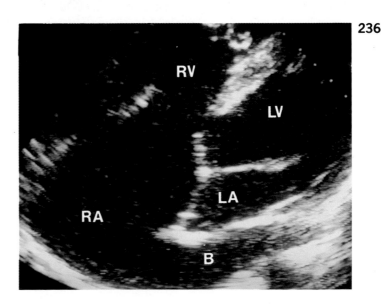

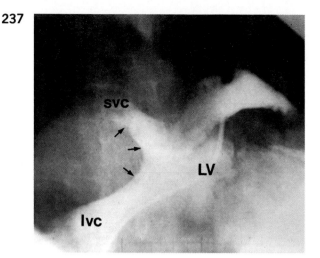

237 Angiogram (antero-posterior projection) in a patient with Mustard repair of transposition of the great arteries showing the atrial baffle (arrows).

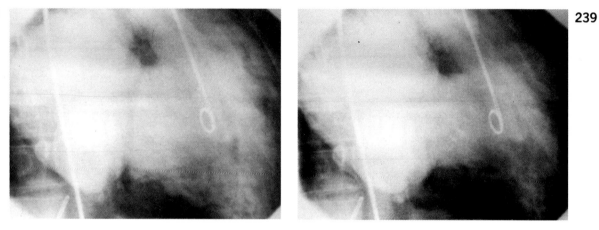

238, 239 Important complications of the Mustard procedure include baffle obstruction to systemic and pulmonary venous return and arrhythmias. In the long term, failure of the systemic ventricle (morphological right ventricle) which is operating at systemic arterial level may occur. Morphological right ventricular angiogram (right anterior oblique projection; systole **238**, diastole **239**) showing a dilated, poorly contracting ventricle with severe tricuspid regurgitation.

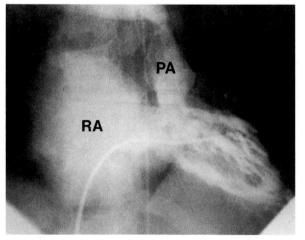

240 Morphological right ventricular angiogram (antero-posterior projection) in Rastelli repair of transposition of the great arteries. Injection of the ventricle shows filling of the Rastelli conduit and pulmonary arteries; there is some tricuspid regurgitation.

Corrected transposition of the great arteries

Corrected transposition of the great arteries is characterized by transposition of the great arteries, with the right atrium connected to the left ventricle through the mitral valve and the left atrium connected to the right ventricle through a tricuspid valve. Therefore, the circulatory pathways are normal and in the absence of common associated lesions, such as ventricular septal defect and pulmonary stenosis, there may be no apparent cardiac abnormality. In such patients, complete heart block and tachyarrhythmias may be the presenting features in adult life. Also in late adult life, failure of the right ventricle, which is carrying the systemic circulation, may occur.

The physical signs are not diagnostic, though there may be a loud second heart sound, since the aorta lies anterior, and evidence of associated congenital heart lesions can be detected. Electrocardiography shows reversal of the normal Q wave pattern with Q waves in leads II and a VR and with QS complexes in V3, a VF and precordial leads. The chest radiograph may show an abnormal position of the aortic arch, but echocardiography and ventriculography may be necessary to make a complete morphological diagnosis.

241 Long axis section of the heart showing an anteriorly placed aortic valve and a posterior stenosed pulmonary valve. There is a large ventricular septal defect connecting the anteriorly placed right ventricle with the posteriorly placed left ventricle.

242 Phonocardiogram and jugular venous pressure in corrected transposition. There is a loud systolic murmur arising from the ventricular septal defect and cannon 'a' waves in the venous pressure from the complete heart block.

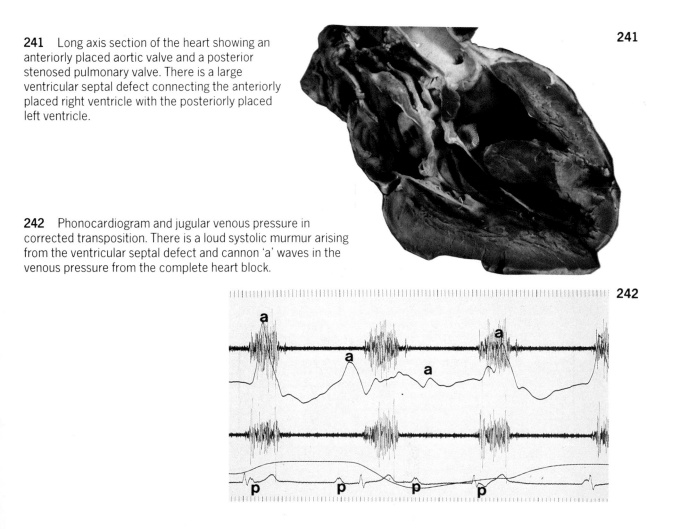

241

242

243

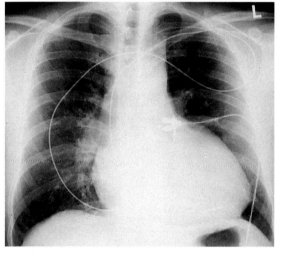

243 Corrected transposition is associated with brady- and tachyarrythmias. This electrocardiogram shows the development of complete atrioventricular block in a patient with corrected transposition.

244

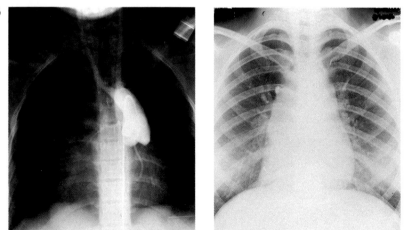

244, 245 Chest radiograph in corrected transposition typically shows an unusually narrow waist and there may be cardiomegaly, particularly if there is an associated ventricular septal defect (**244**). A right-sided aortic arch is a common associated feature in corrected transposition and is evident on the chest radiograph (**245**)(right hand panel) or seen on angiography (**245**)(left hand panel).

245

246   Cross-sectional echocardiography (apical four chamber view) in corrected transposition with the morphological left ventricle seen on the right with its usual smooth appearance. The morphological right ventricle has heavily trabeculated endothelial surfaces and is seen on the left.

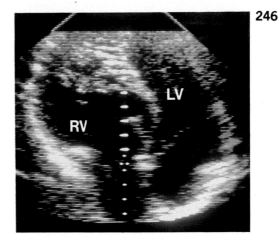

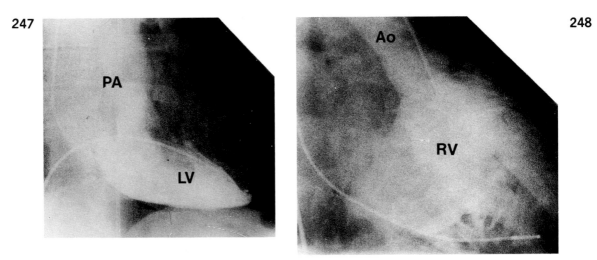

247, 248   Ventriculograms is corrected transposition. The systemic venous ventricle has a smooth appearance and the shape of a morphological left ventricle (**247**). The pulmonary artery can be seen filling from this injection. An arterial catheter, passed retrogradely through the aortic valve, fills a dilated and heavily trabeculated cavity which is the morphological right ventricle (**248**). There is also left atrioventricular valve regurgitation. A pacemaker is present within the morphological left ventricle because the patient had complete heart block.

Double outlet right ventricle/ double outlet left ventricle

Double outlet right ventricle is a condition in which the aorta and pulmonary arteries arise wholly or in great part from the right ventricle with an associated ventricular septal defect. It should be distinguished from transposition of the great arteries with ventricular septal defect and Fallot's tetralogy. The condition is rare and the natural history is indistinguishable from Fallot's tetralogy or pulmonary atresia.

Double outlet left ventricle is an extremely rare condition where both great arteries arise from the left ventricle and again there is an associated ventricular septal defect. The natural history is similar to that of patients with isolated large ventricular septal defects, except in the presence of pulmonary stenosis when it resembles that of Fallot's tetralogy.

249

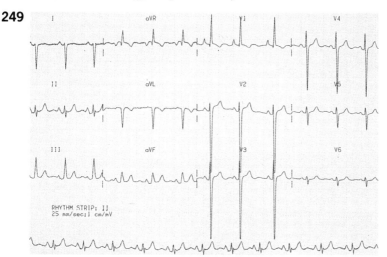

249 Electrocardiogram in double outlet ventricle will show right ventricular hypertrophy; there is also right atrial hypertrophy.

250

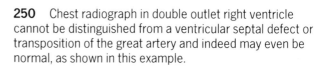

250 Chest radiograph in double outlet right ventricle cannot be distinguished from a ventricular septal defect or transposition of the great artery and indeed may even be normal, as shown in this example.

251, 252 Right ventricular angiogram (antero-posterior projection **251**; lateral projection **252**) showing the aorta and pulmonary artery filling from the right ventricle.

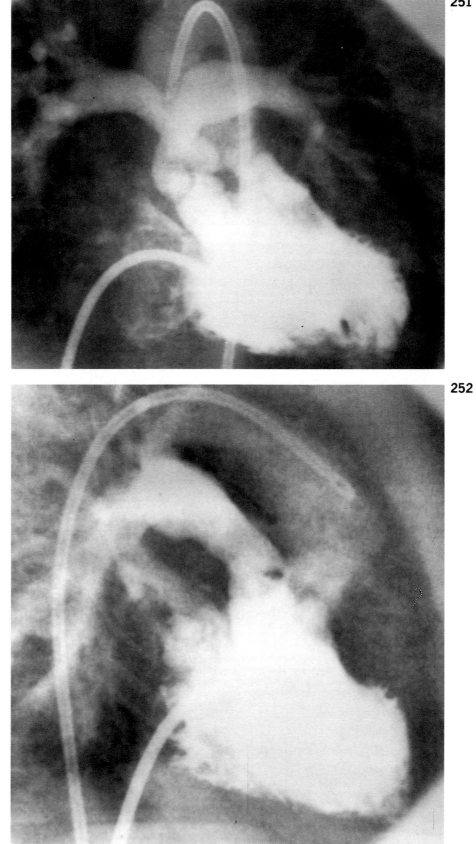

251

252

253

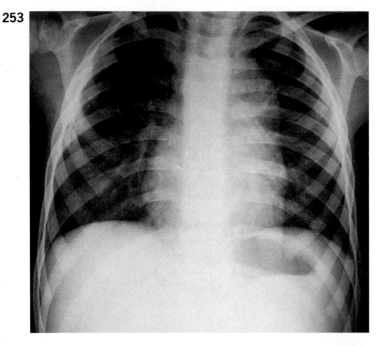

253 Chest radiograph in double outlet left ventricle showing a normal-sized heart.

255

254

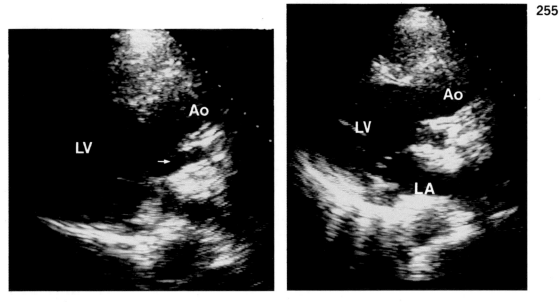

254, 255 Cross-sectional echocardiogram in double outlet left ventricle with pulmonary stenosis in systole (**254**) and diastole (**255**). The aorta (Ao) is shown anteriorly and a stenotic pulmonary artery (arrow) can be seen rising posteriorly from the same ventricular cavity.

Arteriovenous fistula

Arteriovenous fistulae are rare conditions in which a communication is present in either the systemic or pulmonary circulation. Pulmonary fistulae, if large, may lead to cyanosis or heart failure and systemic fistulae, again if large, can lead to heart failure. Although these fistulae may be evident on the plain chest radiograph, they are best demonstrated by angiography.

256, 257 Chest radiograph in a left aorto-pulmonary fistula showing abnormal shadowing in the left upper zone (**256**) which is demonstrated to be a fistula (arrow) on aortography (**257**).

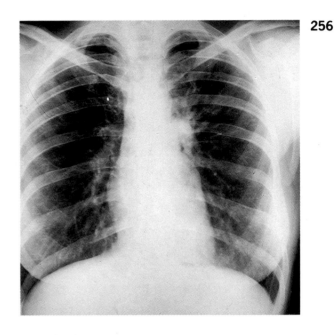

256

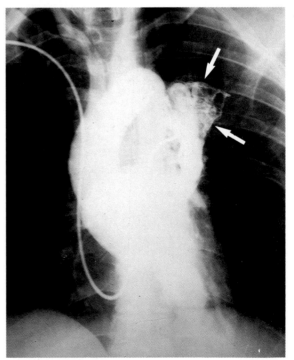

257

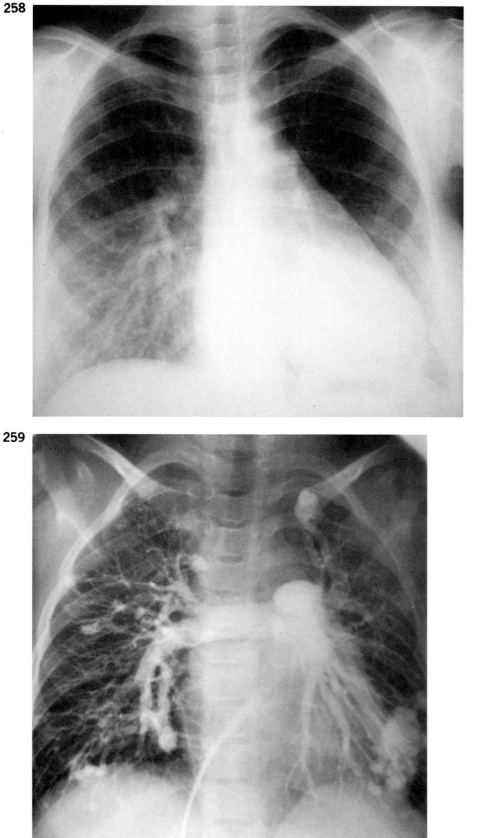

258

259

258, 259 Chest radiograph in a patient with multiple arteriovenous fistulae showing shadowing in the right lower zone and cardiomegaly (**258**). Pulmonary arteriography shows multiple arteriovenous fistulae (**259**). The cardiomegaly is due to the large left to right shunt.

Aortic valve stenosis

Congenital abnormalities of the aortic valve are very common and largely consist of a bicuspid aortic valve, though occasionally, the aortic valve may have no commissures (acommissural) or one commissure (unicommissural). Very occasionally, three cuspid valves may be congenitally stenotic. Congenital aortic stenosis is more common in men than in women. Severe aortic valve stenosis presents in neonatal life with heart failure and death. Sudden death may be a form of presentation in older children; in adults, angina, heart failure and arrhythmias can occur. In children with deformed, non-stenotic aortic valves, only 10 per cent will progress to more severe forms of aortic stenosis. The classical auscultatory features of a congenital bicuspid aortic valve

are an early ejection click and a quiet systolic murmur; with the development of aortic stenosis, the murmur becomes loud and long and the pulse is slow rising. The click will be maintained even in severe aortic stenosis and even when the valve is predominantly regurgitant. In older patients degeneration and calcification of the valve occur; the click will then no longer be present. The electrocardiogram and chest radiograph will show left ventricular hypertrophy which may be confirmed by echocardiography. Cross-sectional echocardiography may be used to demonstrate the morphology of the valve and Doppler echocardiography can be used to assess the gradient across the valve.

Non-stenotic bicuspid valve

260

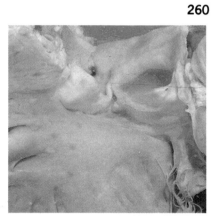

261

262

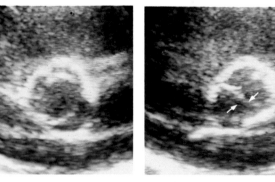

260—262 Opened aorta showing a non-stenotic congenital bicuspid valve (**260**). Auscultation will show an early ejection click (x) and a quiet systolic murmur (**261**). Cross-sectional echocardiogram (parasternal short axis view) in systole (left) and diastole (right) shows a bicuspid (arrowed) non-stenotic aortic valve (**262**).

263

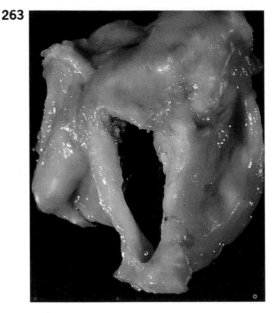

264

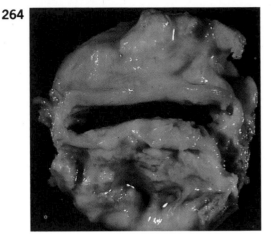

263 Excised aortic valve which is unicuspid. Unicuspid aortic valves may have no commissures (acommissural) or have one commissure like this valve (unicommissural). This valve has severe focal thickening with heavy calcific deposits, particularly along the line of the commissure and the orific is severely stenotic.

264 Excised bicuspid aortic valve removed from a 72-year-old man. The gradient across the valve was 130 mm Hg. The commissures are aligned in a left to right distribution and the cusps are heavily calcified and immobile.

265

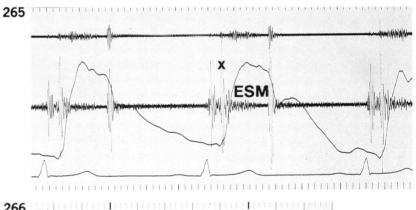

266

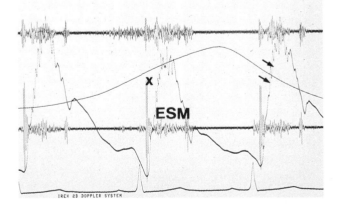

265, 266 In mild congenital aortic stenosis there will be an ejection click and a quiet systolic murmur without a slow rising pulse (**265**). In contrast, in severe congenital aortic stenosis, there is a loud ejection systolic murmur with persistence of the click and the pulse is slow rising (arrow) (**266**).

267 Electrocardiogram in aortic valve stenosis will show left ventricular hypertrophy, most evident in the limb leads.

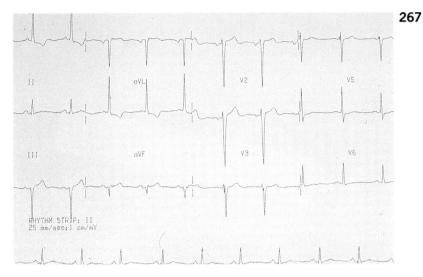

268 Chest radiograph in congenital aortic valve stenosis shows ventricular hypertrophy and a dilated ascending aorta.

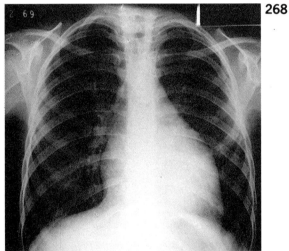

269 Chest radiograph (lateral projection) showing calcification (arrow) in the aortic area.

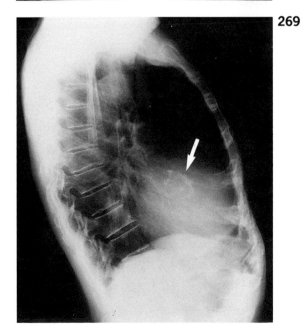

270

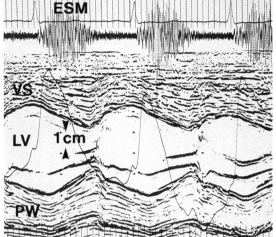

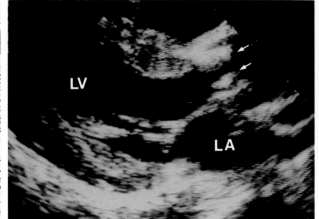

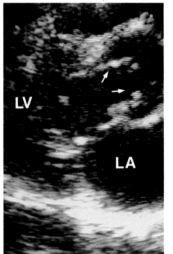

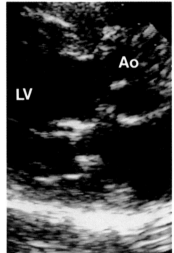

272

270—272 Echocardiography in aortic stenosis. M-mode echocardiogram in severe valvular aortic stenosis shows marked left ventricular hypertrophy and the phonocardiogram shows a loud ejection systolic murmur (**270**). Cross-sectional echocardiography (parasternal long axis view) confirms the presence of left ventricular hypertrophy and shows thickening of the aortic valve (arrowed) which is immobile (**271**). Bicuspid aortic valve may dome (arrow) in systole (**272**) (systole right hand image, diastole left hand image).

273

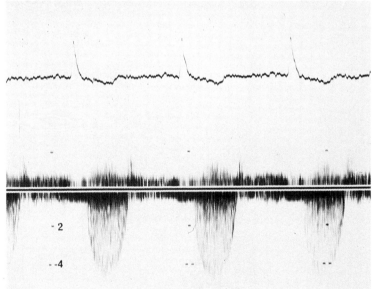

273 Apical continuous wave Doppler showing the severity of valvular aortic stenosis. In this example, the gradient across the aortic valve is approximately 4m/s equating to an aortic valve gradient of over 60 mm Hg.

274 Magnetic resonance scan in aortic stenosis showing a grossly hypertrophied left ventricle (diastole left, systole right).

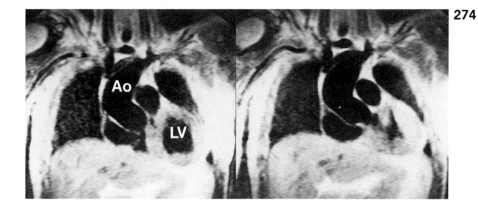

275 Haemodynamic tracing in aortic valve stenosis showing a large gradient between the left ventricle and femoral artery.

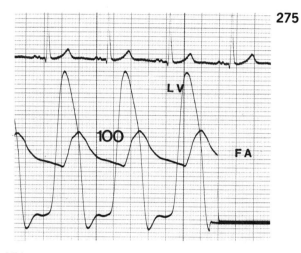

276

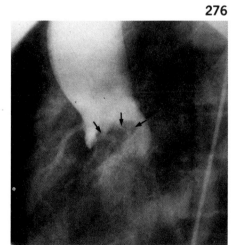

276, 277 Aortogram (left anterior oblique projection; systole **276**, diastole **277**) showing a domed stenosed bicuspid aortic valve (arrowed).

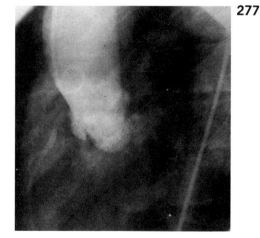

278

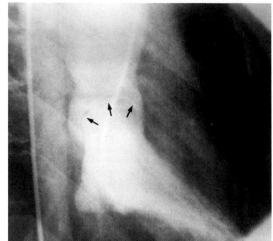

278 Left ventriculogram (right anterior oblique projection) showing severe hypertrophy and a domed aortic valve (arrow).

279

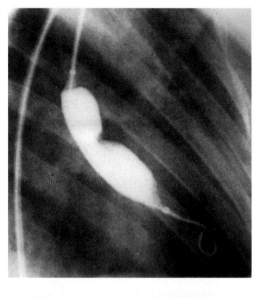

280

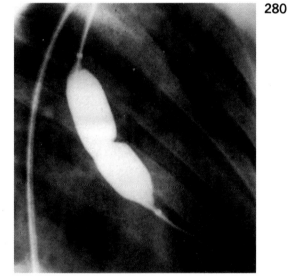

281

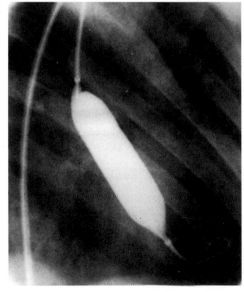

279—281 Balloon aortic valvotomy. A balloon catheter has been passed retrogradely across the aortic valve from the femoral artery. On initial inflation there is wasting of the balloon at the region of the stenosis (**279**), but following dilatation there is progressive inflation of the balloon (**280, 281**).

Subvalvular aortic stenosis

Subvalvular aortic stenosis is caused by obstruction beneath the aortic valve due to discrete fibrous or fibromuscular ridge or a longer fibromuscular tunnel. This condition needs to be differentiated from hypertrophic cardiomyopathy. It may occur as a component of other congenital anomalies such as coarctation of the aorta, ventricular septal defect or abnormalities of the mitral valve. Subvalvular aortic stenosis is less common than valvular obstruction and tends to present late in infancy or in adult life. The presentation is similar to valvular aortic stenosis and the clinical signs are similar to hypertrophic cardiomyopathy. Subaortic obstruction may be demonstrated on cross-sectional echocardiography or angiography.

282 Left ventricle to show a muscular bulge encroaching on the left ventricular outflow tract causing subvalvular aortic stenosis.

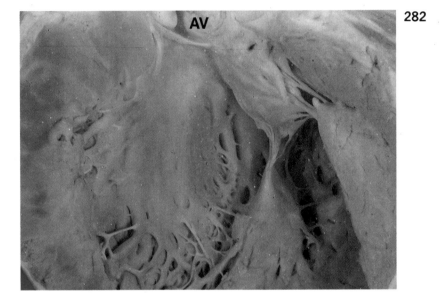

283 Auscultation will reveal an ejection systolic murmur, without a systolic click, with a normal or delayed aortic component of the second heart sound. There is often an early diastolic murmur due to the jet interfering with aortic function. The pulse is usually brisk.

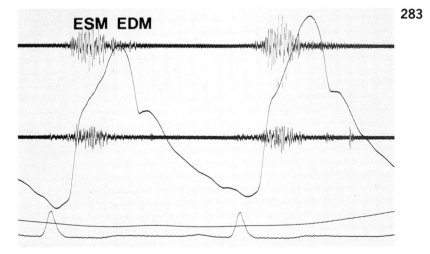

284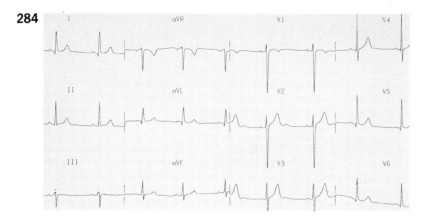

284 The electrocardiogram in subvalvular aortic stenosis will show left ventricular hypertrophy.

285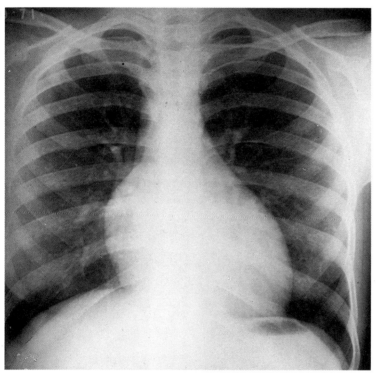

285 Chest radiograph in subvalvular aortic stenosis will show a left ventricular configuration without dilatation of the ascending aorta.

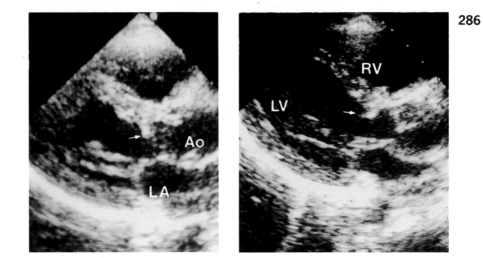

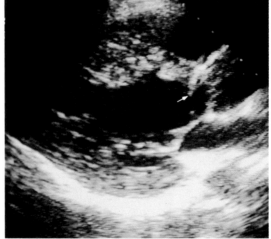

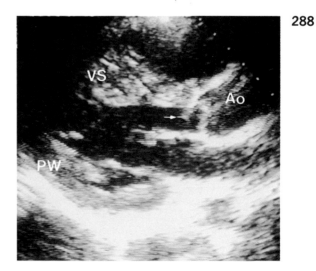

286—288 Cross-sectional echocardiograms (parasternal long axis view) showing a membraneous subaortic obstruction (arrowed) which moves in the cardiac cycle (**286**; systole left, diastole right). In patients with fixed subaortic stenosis there will be marked left ventricular hypertrophy, particularly involving the interventricular septum (systole **287**, diastole **288**).

289

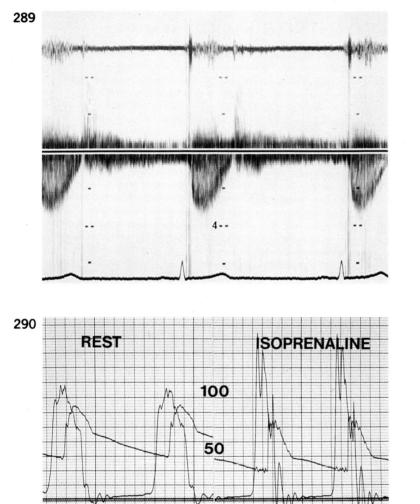

289 Doppler ultrasound in subaortic stenosis showing a peak velocity between 3 and 4 m/s representing significant stenosis. There is also mild aortic regurgitation.

290

REST   ISOPRENALINE

100

50

290 Haemodynamic tracing in subvalvular aortic stenosis will often show a rather small gradient between the left ventricle and aorta at rest, but following isoprenaline, there is marked accentuation of the gradient.

291

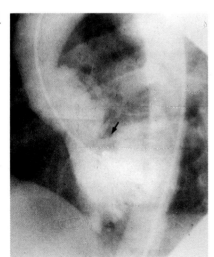

291 Left ventricular angiogram (left anterior oblique cranial projection) showing a muscular bulge (arrow) below the aortic valve.

Supravalve aortic stenosis

Supravalve aortic stenosis is due to obstruction caused by localized or diffuse narrowing of the aorta immediately above the valve. This is the least common congenital type of aortic stenosis and there is a strong association with hypercalcaemia of infancy (William's syndrome). Sudden death can occur at all ages and the prognosis is worse in those patients who have hypercalcaemia of infancy. Few patients reach adult life without corrective surgery. The classical physical sign is the disparity between the right and left carotid pulses, because the high velocity aortic jet may be directed into either carotid artery. The diagnosis may be made on cross-sectional echocardiography or angiography.

292, 293 Classically, supravalve aortic stenosis is associated with hypercalcaemia of infancy (William's syndrome) characterized by a typical elfin facies (**292**) with short little fingers (**293**).

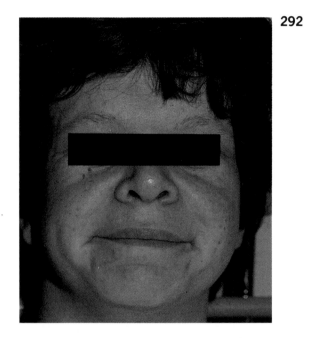

292

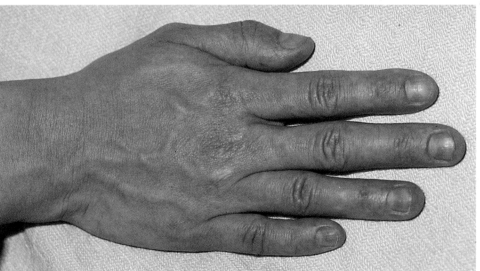

293

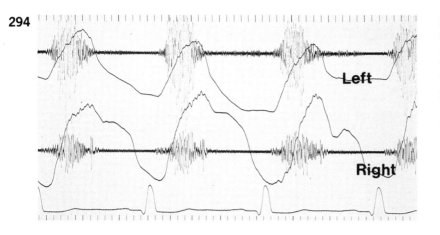

294

294 Physical examination in supravalve aortic stenosis will reveal a disparity in the upstroke of the left and right carotid pulses. In this example, the right carotid is slow rising but the left is very slow rising. There will be a systolic ejection murmur with a loud aortic closure sound and no click.

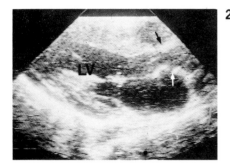

295

295 Cross-sectional echocardiogram (parasternal long axis view) in supravalve aortic stenosis (arrow) showing a waist (arrowed) above the aortic valve.

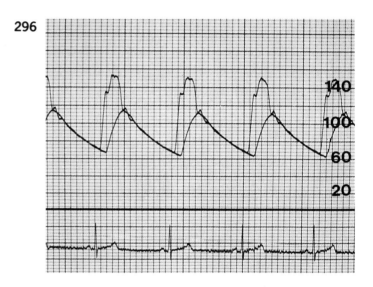

296

296 Haemodynamic tracing in supravalve aortic stenosis will show an intra-aortic gradient.

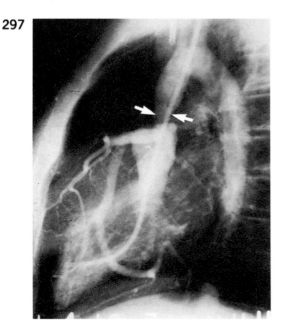

297

297 Left ventricular angiogram (lateral projection) showing supravalvular narrowing (arrowed) above the coronary arteries.

Aortic regurgitation

Congenital aortic regurgitation may be due to a congenital bicuspid or unicuspid aortic valve caused by prolapse of the free edge of the redundant leaflet. Alternatively, aortic root dilatation, due to the Marfan syndrome or similar connective tissue diseases, may lead to aortic regurgitation with an otherwise essentially normal aortic valve. Aortic regurgitation in patients with a bicuspid aortic valve may or may not be associated with aortic stenosis. Mild or moderate aortic regurgitation will have little effect on life expectancy; it is only if aortic regurgitation is severe or becomes severe, due to endocarditis, that left ventricular dilatation and heart failure ensue. Most patients will be asymptomatic until left ventricular dilatation occurs.

The physical signs are those of an early diastolic murmur and a collapsing pulse and there will be left ventricular hypertrophy on the electrocardiogram, chest radiograph and cross-sectional echocardiogram.

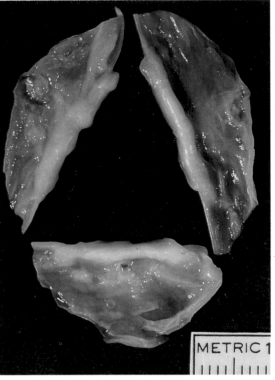

298

298 Excised three cuspid aortic valve in severe aortic regurgitation caused by disease of the aortic root. Each of the cusps is thin, delicate and mobile, similar to a normal valve. There is only slight thickening of the three edges caused by the regurgitant jet.

299—304 The clinical features of Marfan's syndrome include a high arch palate (**299**), . . .

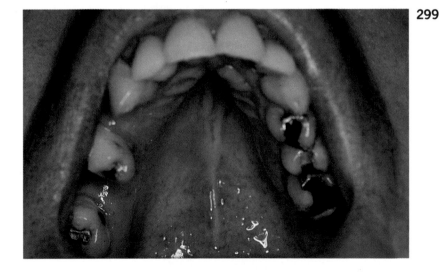

299

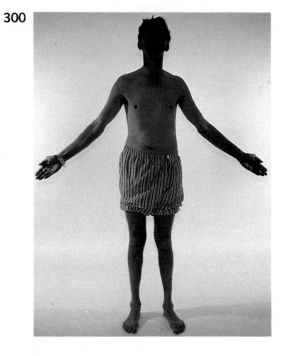

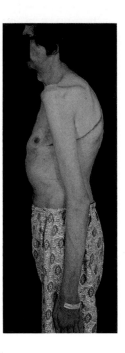

300

302

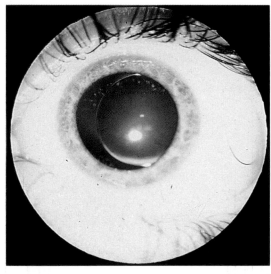

303

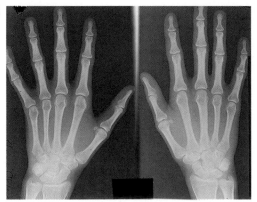

304

. . . a span of the arms greater than the height (**300**), pigeon-chest and kyphoscoliosis (**301**) and posterior dislocation of the lens (**302**). Arachnodactyly (**303**) may be assessed radiographically (**304**).

305 Marfan's syndrome should be distinguished from homocystinuria which may have similar cardiac features and skeletal manifestations. However, the radiograph in patients with homocystinuria will show osteoporosis.

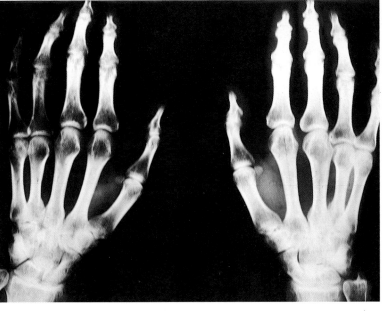

305

306 Aortic regurgitation will show an early diastolic murmur and frequently a systolic ejection flow murmur; aortic closure sound will be normal and pulse collapsing.

306

EDM

307 Electrocardiogram in aortic regurgitation will show evidence of left ventricular hypertrophy and there will be accentuation of the lateral 'q' waves.

307

RHYTHM STRIP: II
25 mm/sec; 1 cm/mV

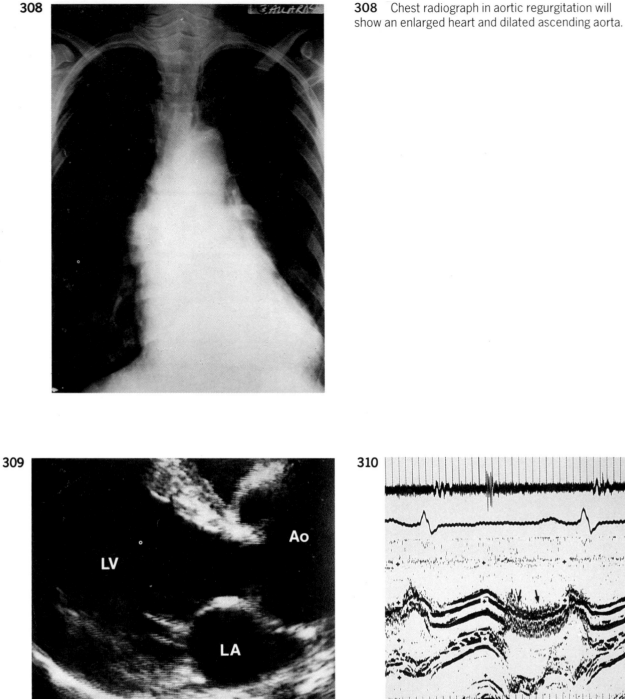

308 Chest radiograph in aortic regurgitation will show an enlarged heart and dilated ascending aorta.

309, 310 Cross-sectional echocardiogram (parasternal long axis view) showing gross dilatation of the ascending aorta in Marfan's syndrome. This has led to dilatation of the aortic valve and severe aortic regurgitation resulting in dilatation of the left ventricle (**309**). Flutter of the anterior leaflet of the mitral valve (arrow) seen on the M-mode echocardiogram (**310**) is a pathognomonic feature of aortic regurgitation.

311, 312 Aortic regurgitation may be demonstrated by Doppler ultrasound even when clinically unapparent. This may be important in patients with aortic root disease. In this example, there is a diastolic jet visualized by continuous wave imaging from the apex across the aortic valve (**311**). Colour flow Doppler shows early (left) and late (right) diastolic jets of aortic regurgitation (**312**).

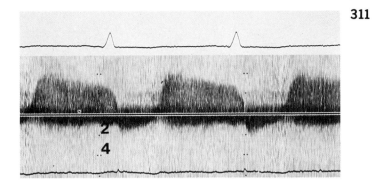

311

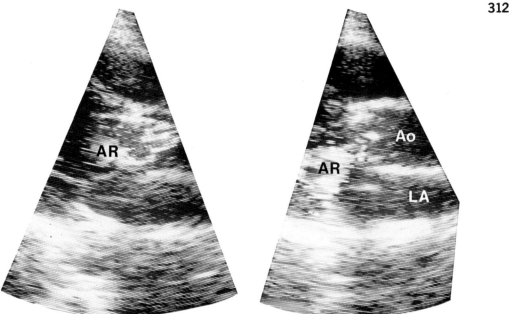

312

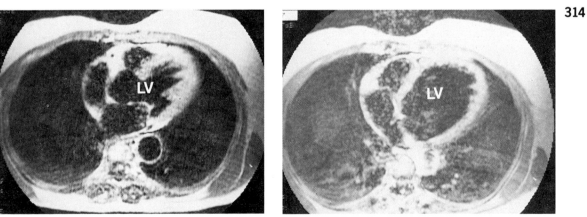

313

314

313, 314 Magnetic resonance scan (systole **313**; diastole **314**) showing a dilated hypertrophied left ventricle in aortic regurgitation.

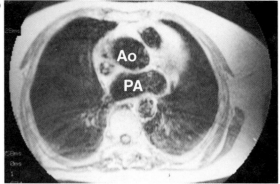

315 Magnetic resonance scan at the level of the pulmonary artery bifurcation showing a dilated ascending aorta.

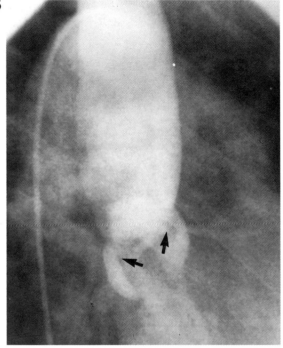

316 Aortogram (lateral projection) showing a bicuspid aortic valve. The left ventricle is filling via the aortic regurgitation.

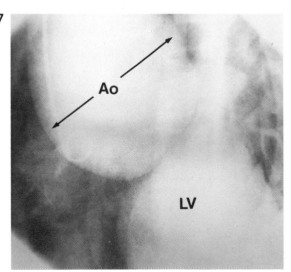

317 Aortogram (left anterior oblique projection) showing a hugely dilated aortic root and ascending aorta in Marfan's syndrome. The left ventricle is again filling via the massive aortic regurgitation.

Aortic dissection

Aortic dissection is a well known complication in patients with Marfan's syndrome. Survival is infrequent without surgical repair and the diagnosis can usually be made by computed tomographic scanning.

318, 319 Aortic sinuses in Marfan's syndrome are large and bulging and prolapse outwards (**318**). The descending aorta shows a dissection; the false channel is larger than the true aortic lumen and it contains no thrombus (**319**).

318

319

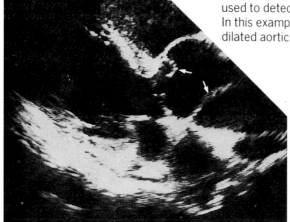

320 Cross-sectional echocardiogram (parasternal long axis view) may be used to detect the presence of a flap (arrows) within the ascending aorta. In this example a flap can be seen anteriorly and posteriorly within a very dilated aortic root.

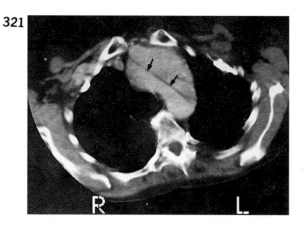

321 Computed tomographic scan of aortic dissection. A flap (arrow) can be seen across the arch of the aorta.

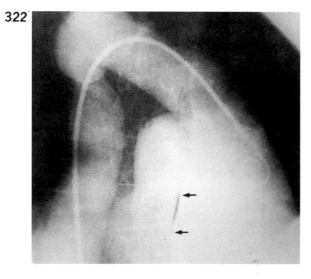

322 Aortogram showing dissection of the ascending aorta (Ao) with false aneurysm formation. Contrast has been injected into the anterior false lumen and the flap (arrow) separating this from the true lumen can be seen (arrows).

Mitral valve prolapse

Mitral valve prolapse is one of the most common congenital anomalies; more frequent in women than in men and present in up to 5 per cent of all healthy young women. Usually mitral valve prolapse is of no significance, but occasionally it can lead to symptoms such as chest pain or palpitations. Rarely, more severe forms with valve thickening and mitral regurgitation will occur and may lead to significant mitral regurgitation. These patients can also develop rupture of their chordae tendinae which can lead to acute severe regurgitation.

The classical physical signs are those of a systolic click and late systolic murmur. Mitral valve prolapse can be readily demonstrated by cross-sectional echocardiography.

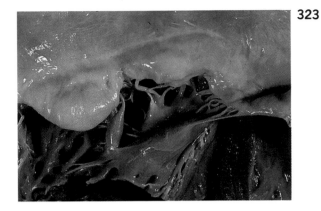

323

323, 324 Floppy, non-regurgitant mitral valve, viewed from the left atrium. There is only a slight increase in surface area with some focal thickening of the leaflets. Excision of a floppy mitral valve (**324**) which was regurgitant; in addition there was rupture of the chordae tendinae.

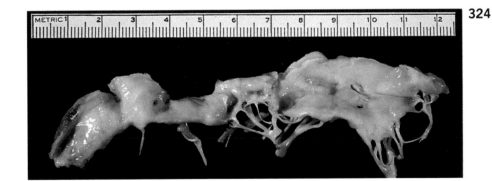

324

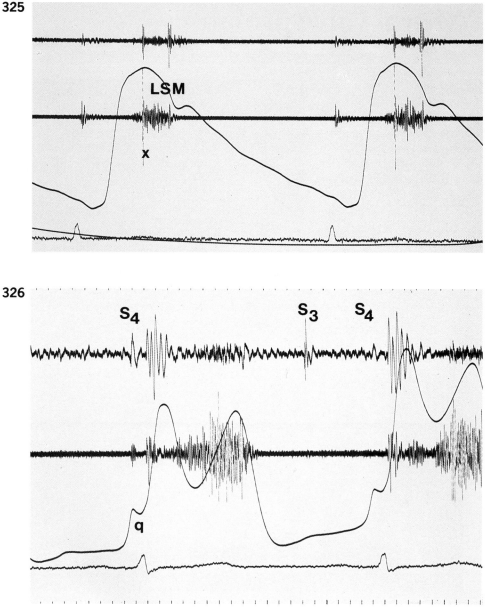

325, 326 Auscultatory features in mitral valve prolapse. Mild mitral valve prolapse is associated with a systolic click (x) and a late systolic murmur (LSM) which is maximally heard at the apex. The pulse is normal (**325**). In severe mitral regurgitation, due to prolapse associated with ruptured chordae, there is a loud pansystolic murmur and third and fourth heart sounds (**326**). The apex shows a tall 'a' wave representing an augmented left atrial component to left ventricular filling.

327, 328 Electrocardiograms in mitral valve prolapse. Mild mitral valve prolapse is often associated with a normal resting electrocardiogram but inferior T wave inversion and extrasystoles can be seen, as in this example (**327**). More severe mitral valve prolapse with mitral regurgitation may show left atrial enlargement (biphasic P wave in V1)(**328**).

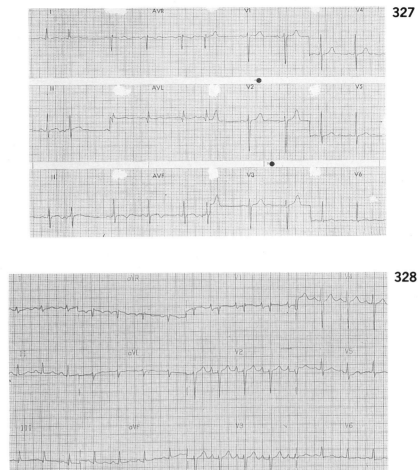

327

328

329 Chest radiograph in mitral valve prolapse may be normal, but when mitral regurgitation is severe, the heart will be enlarged and there will be evidence of pulmonary venous congestion.

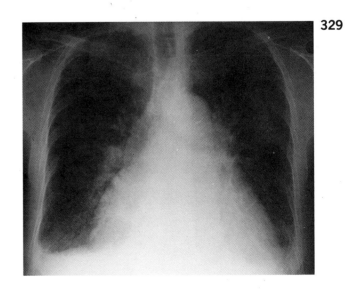

329

111

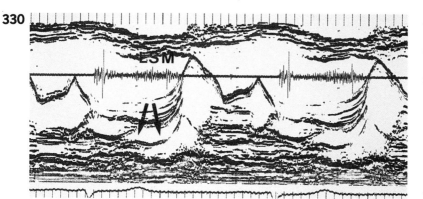

330

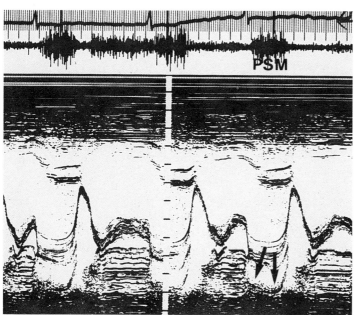

331

330—333 Echocardiograms in mitral valve prolapse. M-mode echocardiogram with simultaneous phonocardiogram showing a late systolic click and murmur coincident with prolapse of the posterior leaflet of the mitral valve (arrows)(**330**). With severe regurgitation, associated with mitral valve prolapse, there is a holosystolic murmur and prolapse of the mitral valve posterior leaflet throughout systole (**331**). Prolapse of one or both leaflets may be demonstrated by cross-sectional echocardiography (**332**) and following rupture of chordae these may be visualized prolapsing into the left atrium during systole (arrow) (**333**).

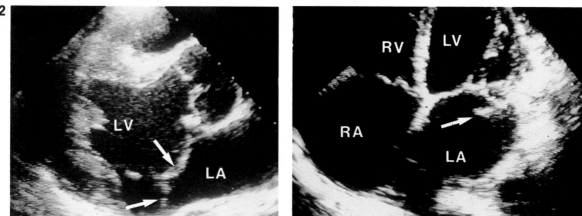

332

333

334 Apical continuous wave Doppler echocardiogram showing holosystolic flow across the mitral valve, representing mitral regurgitation through a floppy valve.

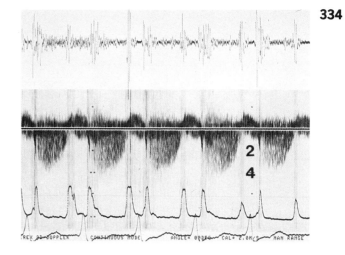

335 Colour flow Doppler echocardiogram (apical long axis view) showing a turbulent jet into the left atrium through an incompetent mitral valve.

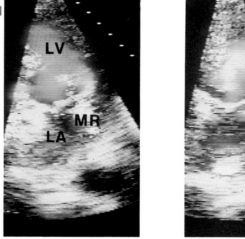
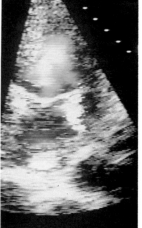

336 Magnetic resonance scan (transverse section) in mitral valve prolapse showing a large left atrium (LA).

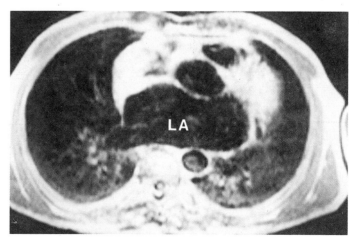

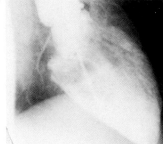
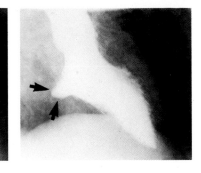

337—339 Left ventricular angiogram (**337**; systole right, diastole left) showing prolapse of the mitral valve (arrowed) without regurgitation. When mitral valve prolapse is severe there will be significant mitral regurgitation and dilatation of the left ventricle (systole **338**; diastole **339**).

339

338

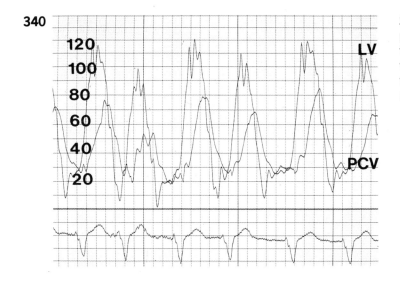

340

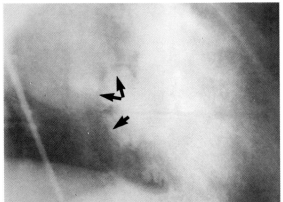

340 Haemodynamic tracing in mitral valve prolapse; if the mitral regurgitation is severe there will be a prominent systolic wave in the wedge tracing without a gradient between left ventricular end-diastolic pressure and wedge pressure.

Cor Triatriatum

Cor Triatriatum is a rare congenital cardiac anomaly in which the pulmonary veins enter the common pulmonary venous chamber, which is located behind the heart and is separated from the true left atrium by a membrane. The presentation and physical signs are similar to congenital mitral stenosis and the diagnosis is made on echocardiography and at cardiac catheterization. The natural history depends on the size of the hole in the membrane communicating between the pulmonary venous chamber and the left atrium; if the hole is small then the presentation will be in early infancy. The natural history is similar to that of mitral stenosis.

341 Left atrium and left ventricle opened to show the membrane (arrow) within the left atrium.

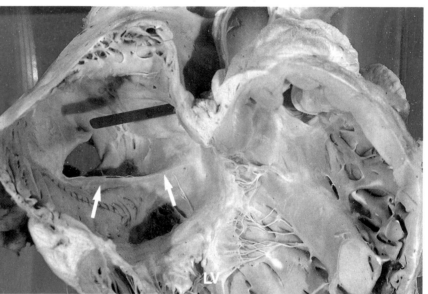

342 Although the clinical picture may resemble mitral stenosis, there may be no murmurs or opening snap, as in this example. The pulmonary component of the second heart sound is loud due to pulmonary hypertension and in this example there is an ejection systolic click (x) from associated mitral valve abnormality.

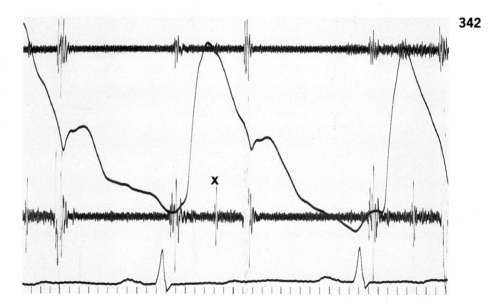

343

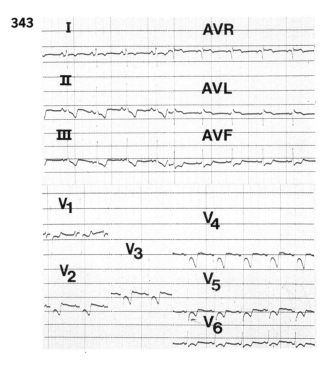

343 The electrocardiogram is similar to congenital mitral stenosis, showing left atrial enlargement.

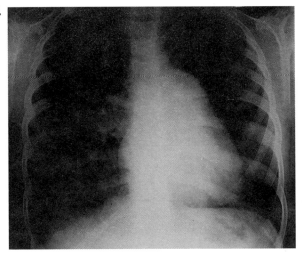

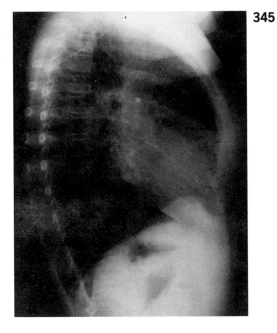

344, 345 Chest radiograph (postero-anterior projection **334**, lateral projection **345**) is also similar to that of congenital mitral stenosis, again showing left atrial enlargement without enlargement of the left atrial appendage. The pulmonary artery is dilated.

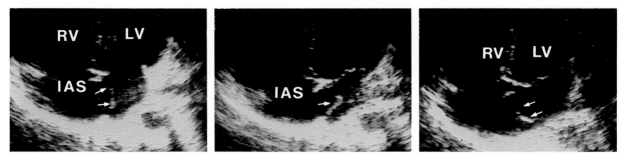

346—348   Cross-sectional echocardiogram in a patient with Cor Triatriatum showing the motion of the inter-atrial septum (IAS) and left atrial membrane (arrow). These can be seen to move throughout the cardiac cycle. The inter-atrial septum is displaced towards the tricuspid valve from the high pressure within the pulmonary chamber.

349   Haemodynamic tracing, which is diagnostic in Cor Triatriatum, showing a large gradient between the left atrium, measured directly, and the pulmonary capillary wedge pressure.

349

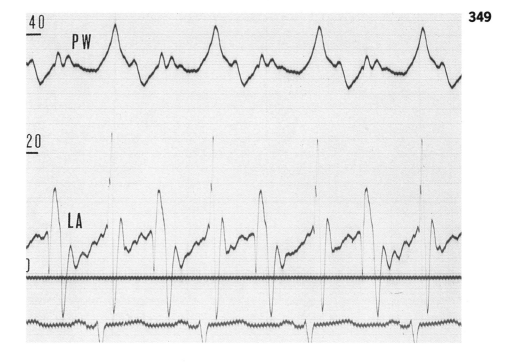

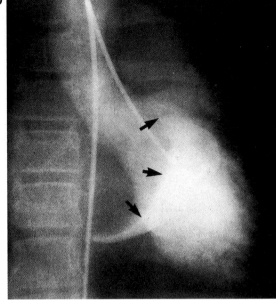

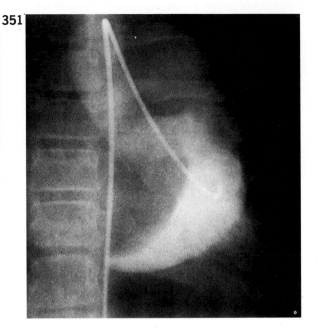

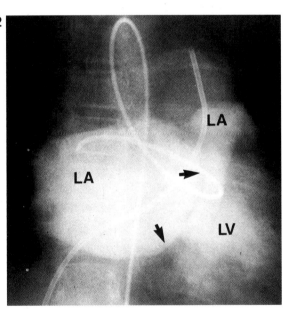

350—352 Left ventricular angiogram (antero-posterior projection; systole **350**, diastole **351**) showing regurgitant contrast filling the lower portion of the left atrium, clearly delineated by the membrane (arrowed). This structure is seen to move throughout the cardiac cycle. Left atrial injection (antero-posterior projection; **352**) showing the upper portion of the left atrium which is dilated; again the membrane is delineated (arrowed) and the lower portion communicates with the left atrial appendage.

Congenital mitral stenosis/mitral atresia

Congenital mitral valve disease is a developmental malformation of one or more of the components of the mitral valve. The mitral orifice may be narrowed by a congenital absence of one or both commissures; this will lead to mitral stenosis of varying severity and is frequently involved with other forms of left-sided heart disease. Congenital mitral stenosis is a rare congenital anomaly with a variable natural history and very few patients survive to adult life without surgery. Mitral atresia usually presents in neonatal life and survival to adult life will depend on the coexisting abnormalities. In adult patients with mitral atresia there is a single ventricle of right ventricular nature. The diagnosis of congenital mitral stenosis and mitral atresia, together with their associated morphological abnormalities, is best made using cross-sectional echocardiography.

353 Cross-sectional echocardiogram (apical long axis view) in congenital mitral stenosis showing a threshold and deformed valve similar to that seen in rheumatic heart disease.

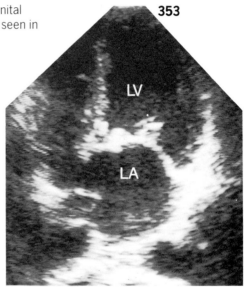

353

354

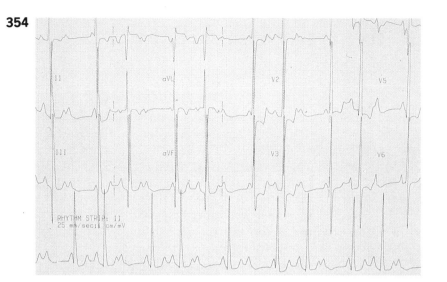

354 Electrocardiogram in mitral atresia showing right ventricular and right atrial hypertrophy.

355

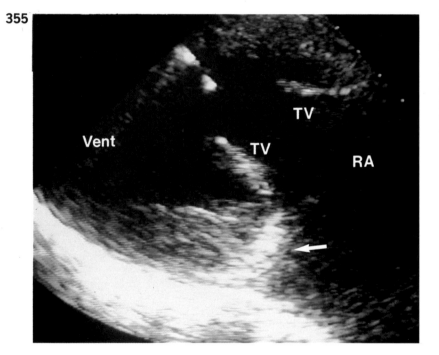

355 Cross-sectional echocardiogram (parasternal long axis view) in mitral atresia. The atretic mitral valve is seen posteriorly as a dense fibrous structure (arrow) beneath which is a muscular chamber representing the atretic left ventricle. The tricuspid valve is large and opens into the main chamber (vent).

Coarctation of the aorta

Coarctation of the aorta is a congenital narrowing of the upper portion of the ascending aorta at the site of the ductus arteriosus. This accounts for approximately 5—8 per cent of congenital heart lesions and as an isolated condition is more common in males than in females. There is an association with Turner's syndrome and less commonly with Noonan's syndrome or congenital rubella. Coarctation of the aorta is frequently associated with more complex forms of congenital heart disease, but in its isolated form it is particularly associated with a bicuspid aortic valve or berianeurysms.

Presentation may be in neonatal life with heart failure, but it may be diagnosed in adults who are completely asymptomatic on a routine examination, particularly for hypertension. The physical signs in the adult are those of hypertension in the upper body and weak, delayed lower limb pulses; collateral murmurs may be present over the back. The chest radiograph will classically show rib notching and the aortic knuckle appears abnormal. The coarctation may be visualized with magnetic resonance imaging or angiography.

In patients presenting in adult life, hypertension, heart failure, endocarditis, aortic rupture and intracranial lesions may develop.

356 Pathological specimen showing coarctation of the aorta.

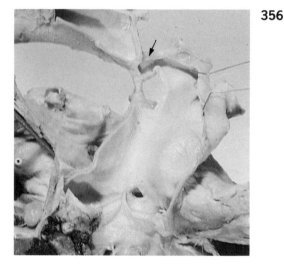

356

357 Retinal photograph showing tortuous vessels in coarctation of the aorta. The retinal changes reflect both the hypertension and also the tortuosity that occurs in the upper limb vessels.

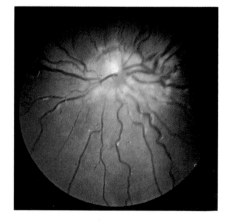

357

358

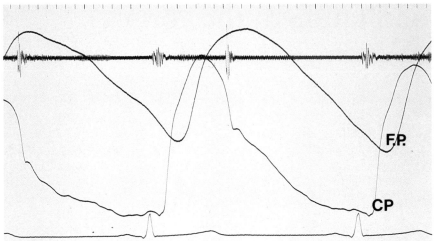

F.P.

CP

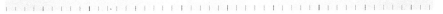

358, 359 Examination of the pulses in coarctation of the aorta will reveal that the femoral pulse, when compared to the carotid, is both delayed and weak (358). On auscultation, murmurs due to collateral blood flow will be heard over the back and evidence of the associated bicuspid valve should be sought with a systolic click and ejection murmur in the aortic area (359).

359

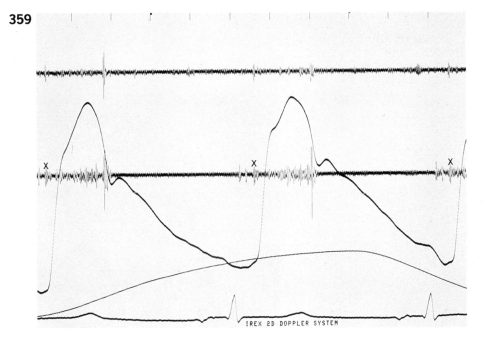

X   X   X

IREX 2D DOPPLER SYSTEM

360 Electrocardiogram in coarctation of the aorta will show left ventricular hypertrophy.

361, 362 A chest radiograph will classically show rib notching (arrow)(**361**). The heart size may be normal or may be enlarged (**361**). Pulmonary oedema occurs as a late phenomoneon as a consequence of both hypertension and associated aortic valve disease (**362**).

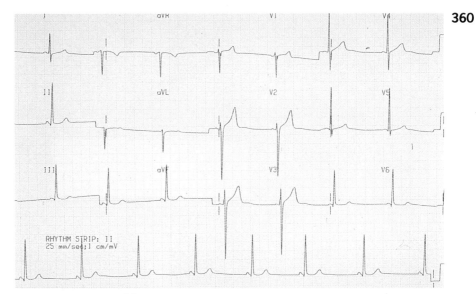

360

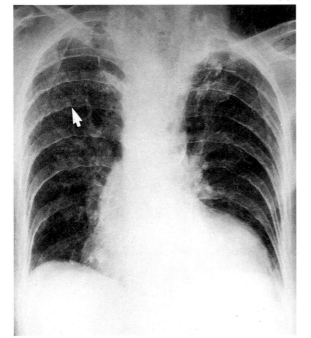

361

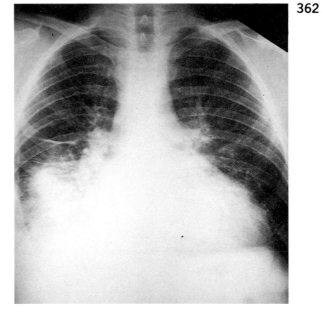

362

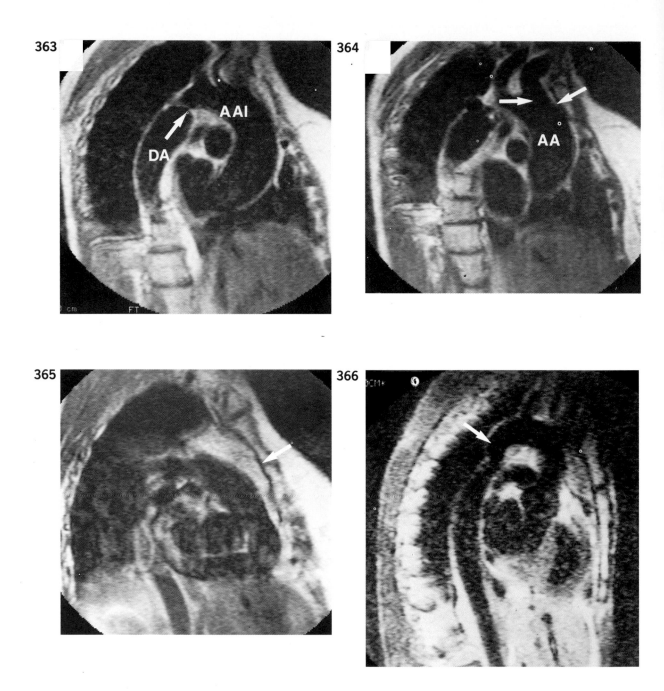

363—366 In the adult, it is usually not possible to demonstrate the coarctation using cross-sectional echocardiography. However, magnetic resonance imaging (transverse sections) will demonstrate the site of obstruction (arrow)(**363**), a dilated ascending aorta (AA) (**364**) and internal mammary artery collaterals (arrow) (**365**). Following repair, there is often residual narrowing (arrow)(**366**).

367 Doppler echocardiography, from the suprasternal notch, may be used to demonstrate the site of obstruction. In the ascending aorta, blood velocity is normal towards the transducer and as the transducer is rotated down the ascending aorta high velocity is seen across the coarctation showing that there is a significant stenosis.

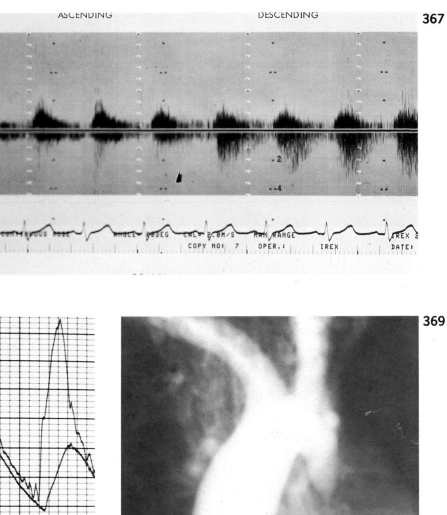

367

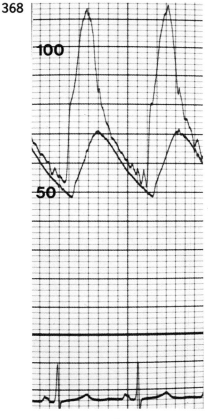

368   Haemodynamic tracing showing the gradient across the coarctation.

369   Aortogram (antero-posterior projection) showing a large ascending aorta and a coarctation distal to the left subclavian.

370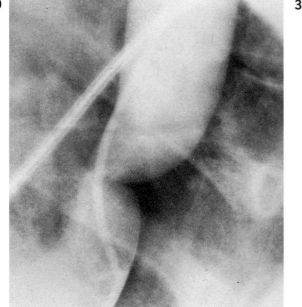

371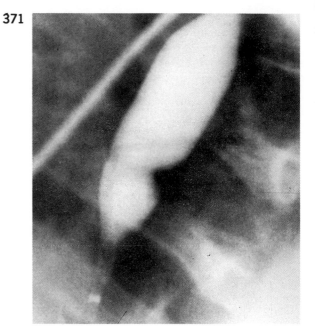

372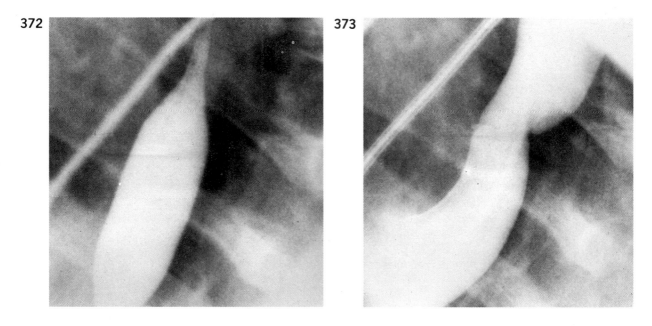

373

370—373 Balloon angioplasty can be performed particularly when a restenosis occurs post-operatively in patients with coarctation of the aorta. Aortogram showing the site of narrowing at the previous anastomosis (right anterior oblique projection **370**). Indentation of the inflated balloon will be caused by the narrowing (**371**) and when the dilatation is complete the balloon fully inflates (**372**). Aortography shows the successful dilatation (**373**).

Sinus of Valsalva aneurysm

Congenital aneurysms of the sinus of Valsalva are thin walled and tubular and nearly always involve the right sinus or adjacent half of the coronary non-sinus. The aneurysms assume clinical importance when they rupture, usually into the right ventricle, but rarely may cause compression or heart block due to the conducting tissue.

Rupture of the sinus of Valsalva aneurysm is an acute event usually causing chest pain and may lead to the development of heart failure, if the shunt is large. The physical signs are characterized by a continuous murmur. A morphological diagnosis can be made using cross-sectional echocardiography or angiography.

374 Excised sinus of Valsalva aneurysm showing the site of rupture into the right ventricle.

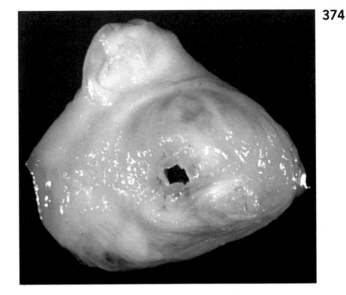

375 The phonocardiogram and carotid pulse show an ejection systolic murmur with intact second heart sound. The lower trace is the left sternal edge phonocardiogram which shows a loud continuous murmur.

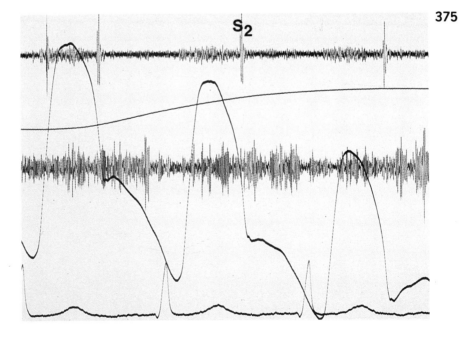

S₂

376 Electrocardiogram in ruptured sinus of Valsalva aneurysm will show left ventricular hypertrophy and there may be bundle branch block deformities (incomplete right bundle branch block in this example) and extrasystoles.

377

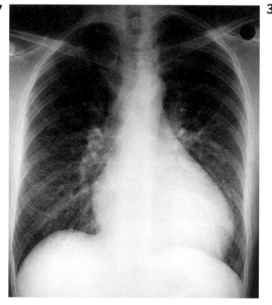

377 Chest radiograph in ruptured sinus of Valsalva aneurysm will show cardiomegaly and there may be pulmonary plethora if the shunt is large.

378

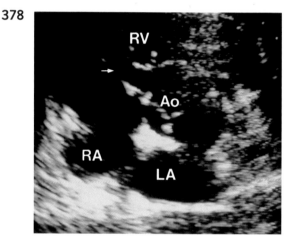

378 Cross-sectional echocardiogram (parasternal short axis view) showing the site of rupture of the sinus of Valsalva aneurysm between the aorta and right ventricle (arrow).

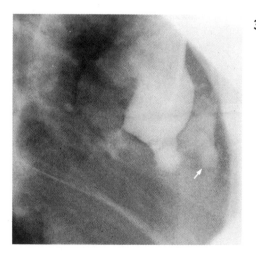

379

379 Aortogram (lateral projection) showing the sinus of Valsalva aneurysm which had ruptured anteriorly into the right ventricle (arrow) with contrast seen in the pulmonary artery.

Hypertrophic cardiomyopathy

Hypertrophic cardiomyopathy is usually transmitted as an autosomal dominant trait, although non-familial cases occur. It is defined as left ventricular hypertrophy of unknown aetiology. The distribution of hypertrophy is characteristically asymmetrical and septal or less commonly symmetrical or predominantly at the apex. The left ventricular cavity is small and there is increased systolic function and impaired diastolic function. The classical physical signs include a jerky pulse, systolic murmur and clinical evidence of left ventricular hypertrophy, including a fourth heart sound. The murmur can be due to either mitral regurgitation or left ventricular outflow tract obstruction. The diagnosis can be made by echocardiography.

Hypertrophic cardiomyopathy can present at any age, from early infancy to even the sixth or seventh decade. It usually presents early in adult life, in many ways, including the detection of an abnormal electrocardiogram or physical signs at a routine examination. Patients may also present with angina, heart failure or palpitations.

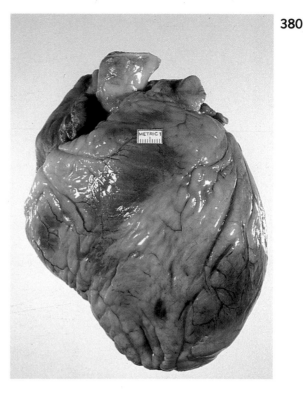

380

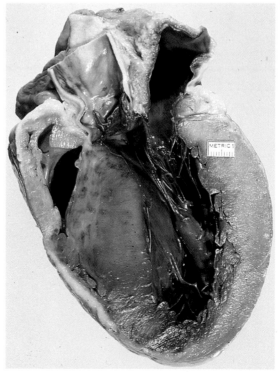

381

380—382 External appearance of the heart in hypertrophic cardiomyopathy. There is marked increase in cardiac weight due to left ventricular hypertrophy (**380**). In the long axis echo view (**381**) there is gross left ventricular hypertrophy, more marked in the septum than in the free wall. Long axis section in hypertrophic cardiomyopathy (**382**); both septum and left ventricular free wall are markedly thickened and the outflow tract is narrow. An area of white thickened endocardium overlies the bulging septum due to contact with the anterior leaflet of the mitral valve (contact lesion).

382

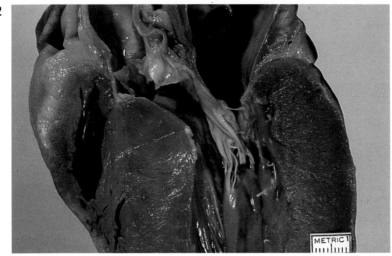

383

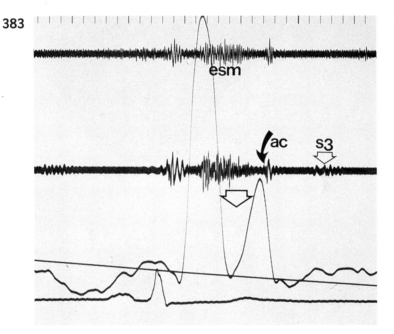

esm

ac   s3

383—385 Physical examination in hypertrophic cardiomyopathy reveals an ejection systolic murmur with delay of aortic valve closure (black arrow) and a third heart sound (S3) is often heard as well as a fourth heart sound (**383**). The pulse is collapsing (broad arrow) due to mid systolic left ventricular outflow obstruction. Figure **384** shows a tall 'a' wave in the apex cardiogram with a sustained systolic wave, representing left ventricular hypertrophy. The Bernheim effect simulates right ventricular hypertrophy and pulmonary stenosis, which is due to the ventricular septum bulging into the right ventricle. The jugular venous pressure shows a tall 'a' wave (**385**).

384

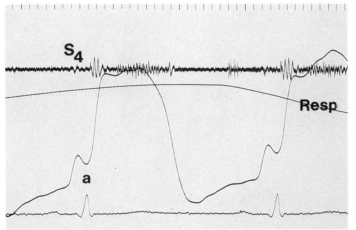

S4

Resp

a

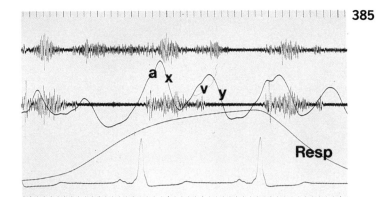

385

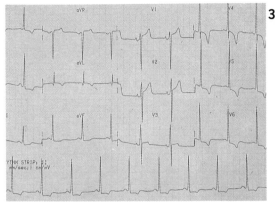

386

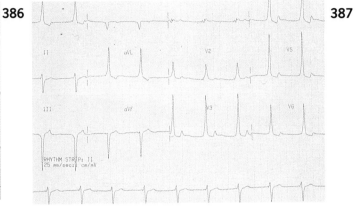

387

386—388 Electrocardiogram in hypertrophic cardiomyopathy will usually show left ventricular hypertrophy with strain (**386**). Occasionally there may be associated pre-excitation syndrome (a short PR interval and delta wave, **387**). In apical hypertrophic cardiomyopathy, left ventricular hypertrophy with strain is often present, but in addition there is deep symmetrical T wave inversion across the mid precordial leads (**388**).

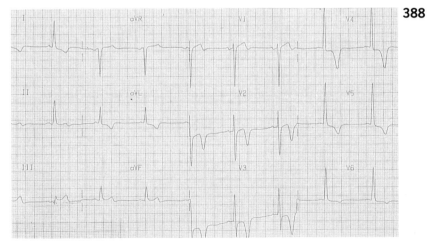

388

389

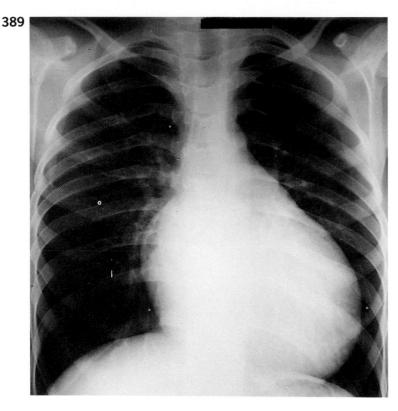

389 Chest radiograph in hypertrophic cardiomyopathy will show left ventricular enlargement.

390

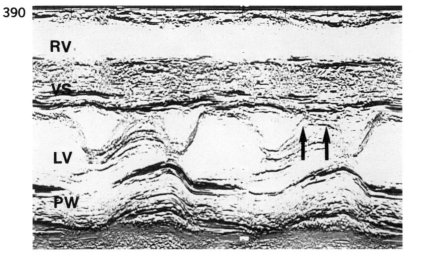

RV

VS

LV

PW

390 M-mode echocardiogram in hypertrophic cardiomyopathy showing asymmetrical septal hypertrophy and systolic anterior motion (arrow) of the mitral valve.

391, 392 Cross-sectional echocardiograms in hypertrophic cardiomyopathy showing gross hypertrophy of the interventricular septum, with a small left ventricular cavity which is eliminated in end-systole (**391**). The hypertrophy of the interventricular septum may be limited just to the left ventricular outflow tract (arrow) (**392**).

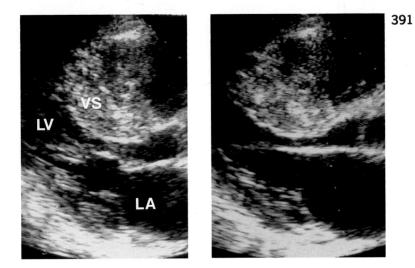

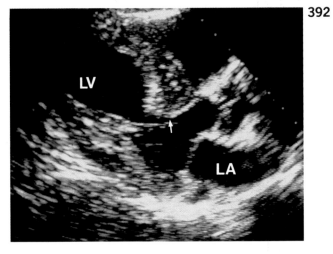

393 Apical hypertrophic cardiomyopathy is a form where the left ventricular hypertrophy is localized to the apex, as in this example.

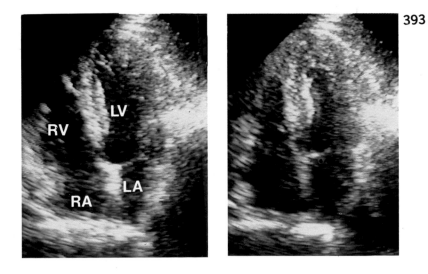

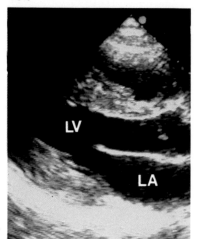

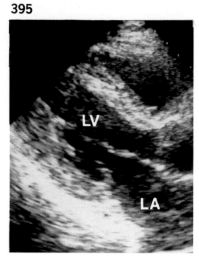

394, 395 In some families with symmetrical hypertrophic cardiomyopathy, the same distribution of left ventricular hypertrophy may be seen in different generations. Figures **394** and **395** show a similar form of hypertrophic cardiomyopathy with symmetrical left ventricular hypertrophy and atrial fibrillation in a father and son, respectively.

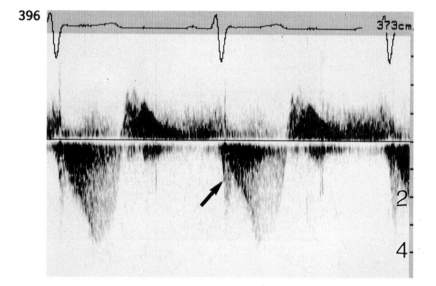

396 Continuous wave Doppler echocardiogram from the apex. Initially, there is a small amount of mitral regurgitation (arrow) and then a slow rising mid systolic gradient from the left ventricular outflow tract obstruction.

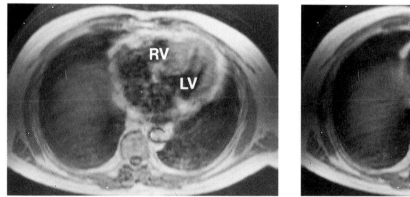

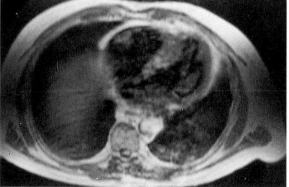

397, 398 Magnetic resonance scan (coronal section) showing (systole **397**; diastole **398**) left ventricular hypertrophy, particularly involving the septum and papillary muscles.

399 Haemodynamic tracing with a resting left ventricular outflow tract gradient and post extrasystolic potentiation (arrow). The pulse is ill-sustained in this condition.

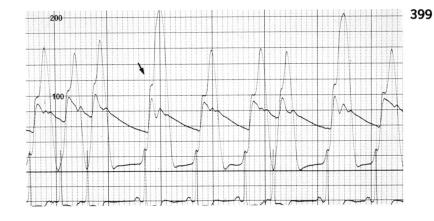

399

400, 401 Left ventricular angiogram in systole (**400**) and diastole (**401**). There is marked deformation of the left ventricular cavity in this right anterior oblique projection, due to the interventricular septum. There is almost complete mid cavity elimination and mitral regurgitation into a large left atrium.

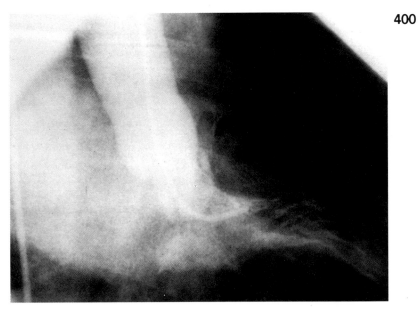

400

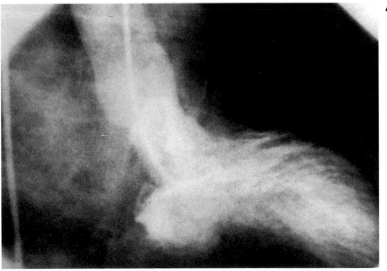

401

Heart muscle disease

Heart muscle disease in adult life is usually due to ischaemic heart disease or dilated cardiomyopathy or follows myocarditis. Very rarely, it may be a congenital abnormality, when there is usually a specific neuromuscular disorder such as limb girdle muscular dystrophy, Friedrich's ataxia, Duchenne's muscular dystrophy, Fabry's disease or mucopolysaccharide disorders. Other than the features of the associated diseases, there are no specific findings in the cardiovascular system that can separate heart muscle disease from any other cause of heart failure.

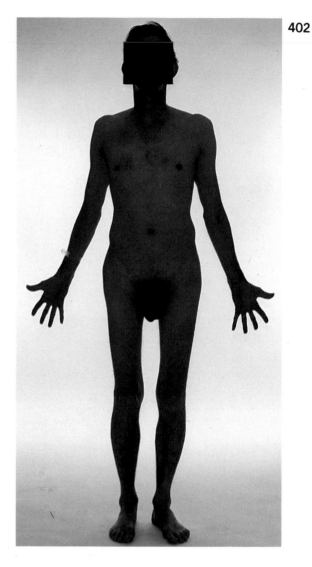

402 Specific neuromuscular disorders, such as limb girdle skeletal myopathy and muscular dystrophy (as in this example), may be associated with heart muscle disease.

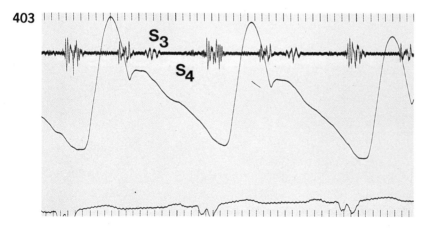

S₃

S₄

403 There are no specific auscultatory features suggestive of heart muscle disease, but rather evidence of heart failure with a third heart sound, a gallop rhythm and an ill-sustained pulse.

404 Electrocardiogram may typically show anterior precordial Q waves or, alternatively, as in this example, left bundle branch block. Atrial fibrillation is a common complication and can lead to clinical deterioration.

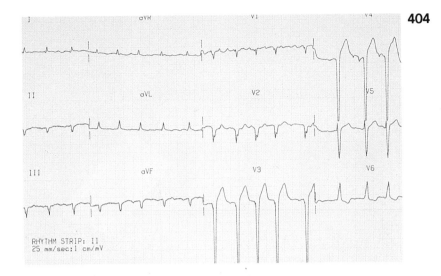

405 Chest radiograph showing cardiomegaly and pulmonary venous congestion.

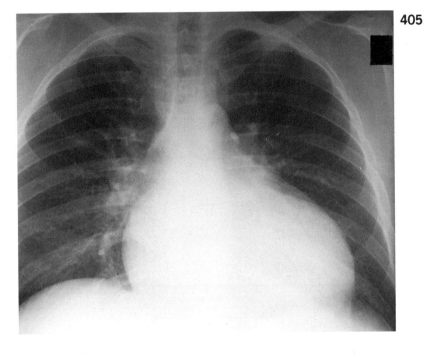

406, 407 Cross-sectional echocardiogram (parasternal long axis view; systole **406**, diastole **407**). The left ventricle is grossly dilated and contracts poorly. There is also left atrial enlargement.

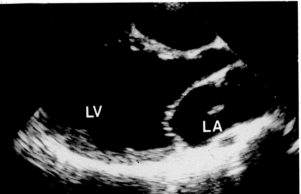

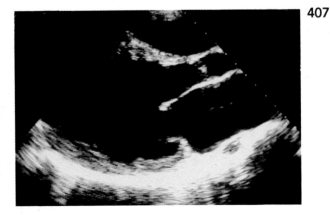

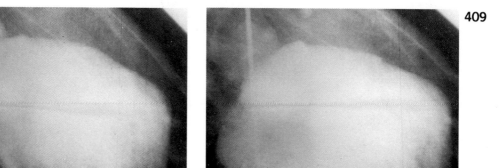

408, 409 Left ventricular angiogram (right anterior oblique projection) showing very poor left ventricular function with a grossly dilated left ventricle (systole **408**, diastole **409**).

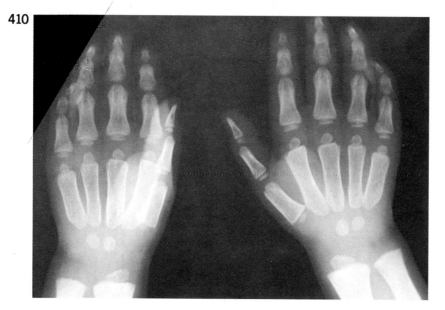

410—412 Rarely, heart-muscle disease may be due to a specific cause such as mucopolysaccharide disease (Hurler's syndrome). Radiograph of the hand will show broad, short phalanges (**410**). The electrocardiogram in Hurler's syndrome will show signs of left ventricular hypertrophy, due to mucopolysaccharide infiltration of the myocardium (**411**), and the chest radiograph will show cardiomegaly and broad spatulate ribs (**412**).

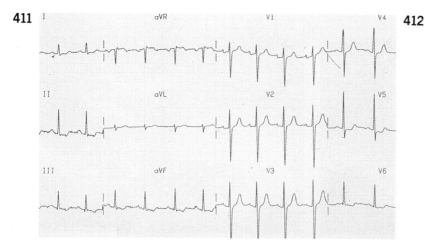

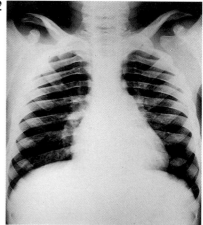

Right ventricular dysplasia

Right ventricular dysplasia or arrhythmogenic right ventricle is a rare congenital heart lesion in which the right ventricle is dilated and dysplastic and usually does not lead to heart failure but causes cardiac arrhythmias. The basic pathological process is the replacement of myocardium with fatty tissue. The diagno-sis is made on cross-sectional echocardiography or angiography. In contrast, Uhl's anomaly produces heart failure and less frequently palpitations and is due to a parchment-like right ventricle and only a few muscle fibres between the epi- and endocardial surfaces.

413, 414 Pathological specimen opened from the right ventricle showing a dilated (**413**), dysplastic and highly trabeculated ventricle (**414**).

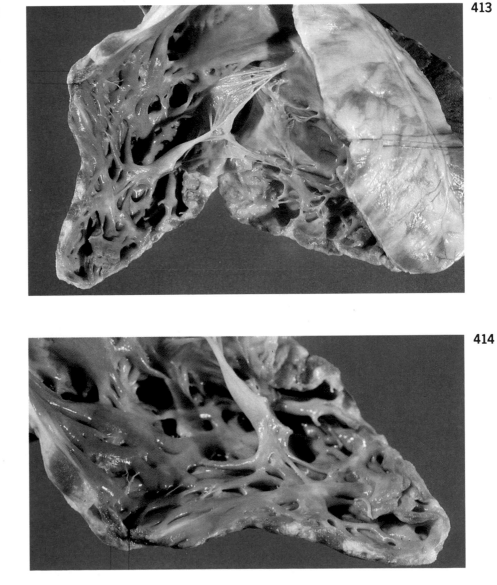

413

414

415

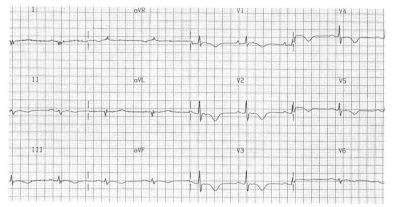

415 Electrocardiogram in right ventricular dysplasia showing right ventricular hypertrophy and T wave inversion across the anterior chest leads.

416

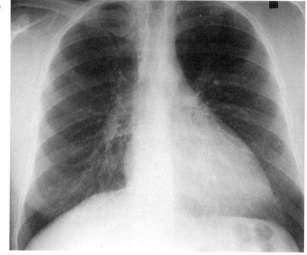

416 Chest radiograph in right ventricular dysplasia will show cardiomegaly which is due predominantly to right ventricular dilatation.

417, 418 Cross-sectional echocardiograms in right ventricular dysplasia. A parasternal long axis view shows a dilated right ventricle and a small left ventricle (**417**). Right ventricular inflow view shows the tricuspid ring to be enlarged and a grossly dilated, poorly functioning right ventricle (**418**).

417

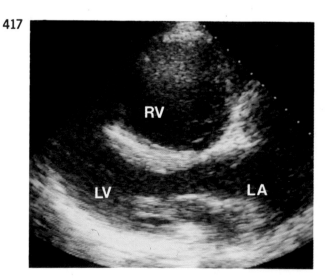

418

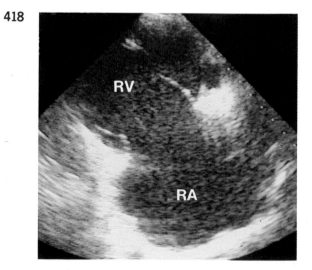

419 The right atrial and right ventricular pressures will equilibrate in right ventricular dysplasia, due to loss of function of the right ventricle.

420, 421 Right ventriculogram (systole **420**, diastole **421**) showing gross dilatation and poor function of the right ventricle.

422 Very rarely, Uhl's anomaly may cause heart failure and palpitations. This is due to thinning and gross dilatation of the so called 'parchment' right ventricle. The chest radiograph shows an enlarged heart, predominantly due to the right atrium and right ventricle.

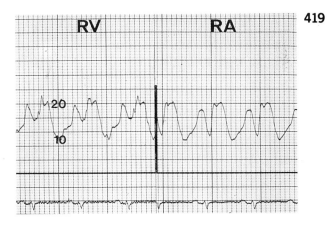

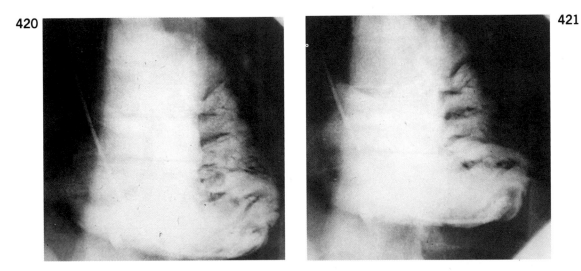

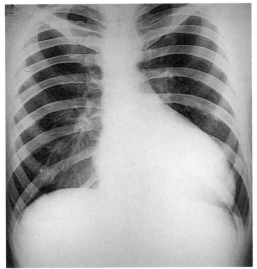

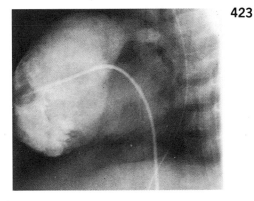

423 Right ventricular angiogram (lateral projection) in Uhl's anomaly showing a dilated and thin right ventricle.

Coronary anomalies

Coronary anomalies usually do not present with symptoms and are found as an incidental finding during coronary angiography. Very occasionally an anomalous coronary artery may be compressed by the pulmonary artery and in these circumstances will lead to angina pectoris. The most serious coronary anomaly is when the coronary artery arises from the pulmonary artery and this may cause angina and acute myocardial infarction presenting in infancy; very rarely patients may present in adult life with these symptoms.

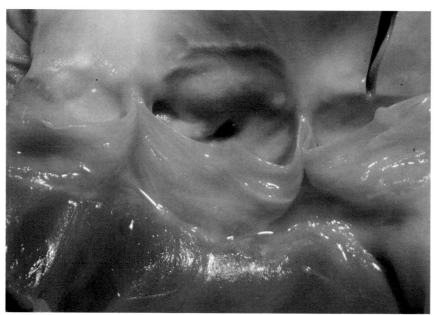

424

424, 425 Macroscopic view of the coronary ostia of a patient in whom the right and left coronary ostia arise from the right coronary artery (**424**); pointers have been inserted into the coronary ostia to show their different courses (**425**).

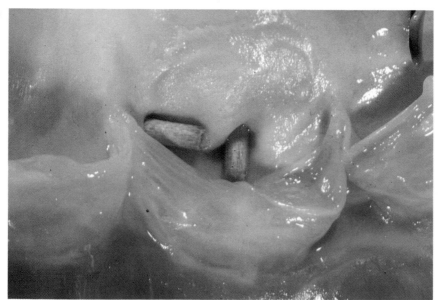

425

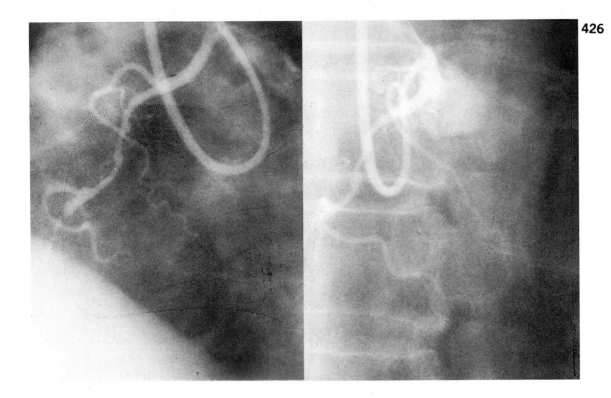

426

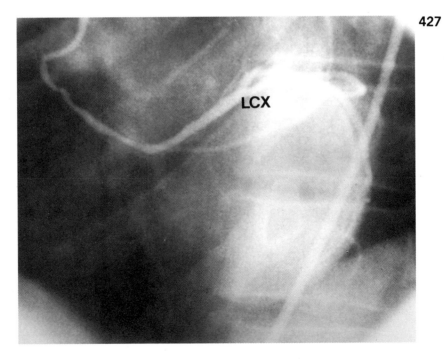

427

LCX

426, 427 Coronary arteries may arise from an anomalous origin. The right coronary artery here arises from the non-coronary sinus (**426**) and the circumflex arises from the right coronary sinus (**427**).

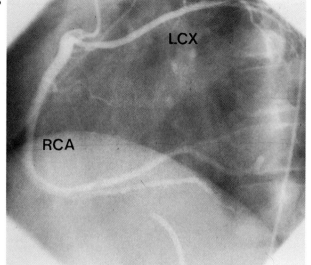

LCX

RCA

428, 429 A coronary artery may arise from another coronary artery. Here the circumflex is arising from the right coronary artery (**428**), the left anterior descending (arrow) from the right coronary (**429**).

429

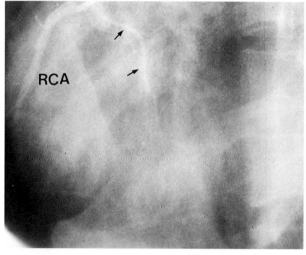

RCA

430

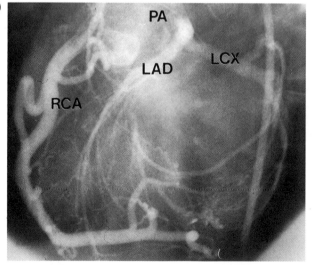

PA

LCX

LAD

RCA

430 The most serious coronary anomaly is when the coronary artery arises from the pulmonary artery and this may often lead to acute myocardial infarction, occurring in infancy. In this example, the left coronary artery arises from the pulmonary artery (left anterior oblique projection). Contrast has been injected into the right coronary artery which fills the left coronary system retrogradely and then fills back into the pulmonary artery.

Infective endocarditis

Infective endocarditis is an important complication of many congenital abnormalities and may convert a mild lesion, such as bicuspid aortic valve, floppy mitral valve or small ventricular septal defects into a severe one. It is still common today in spite of the widespread use of antibiotics and if not- treated energetically and early, patients may die. Often the classical physical signs are not present and the diagnosis rests on the presence of a pyrexia and positive blood cultures in a patient with a cardiac anomaly. Vegetations may be visualized by echocardiography but this is not invariably the case.

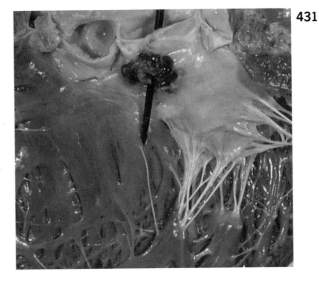

431, 432 Vegetations from infective endocarditis may involve any abnormal cardiac structure such as the aortic valve (**431**) and rarely coarctation of the aorta (**432**).

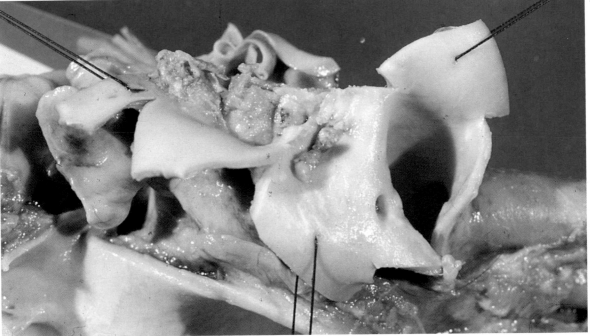

433

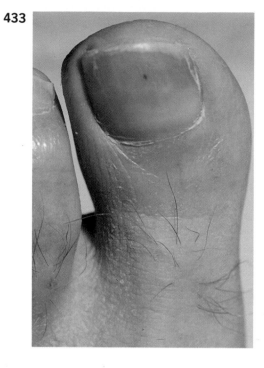

434

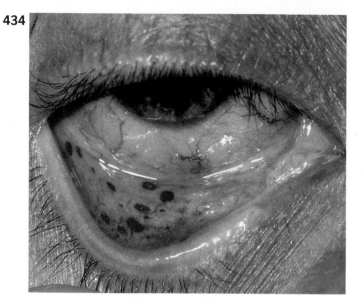

433—436 The pathognomonic physical signs of infective endocarditis include splinter haemorrhages (**433**), sub-conjunctival haemorrhages (**434**), finger clubbing (**435**) and dermal infarcts due to micro-emboli (**436**).

435

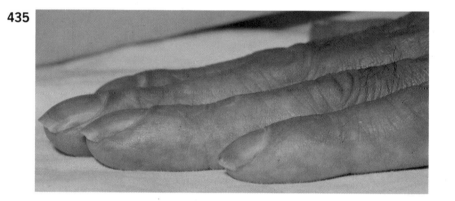

436

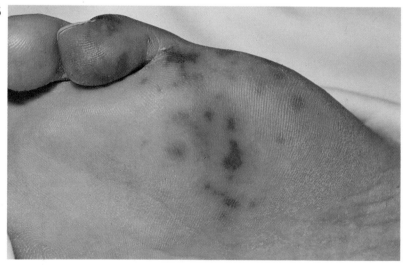

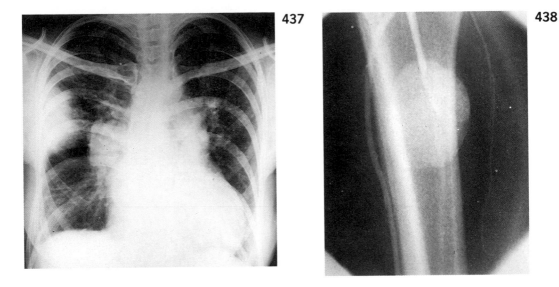

437, 438 Evidence for systemic and pulmonary emboli should be sought. Chest radiograph showing pulmonary infarcts in ventricular septal defect, complicated by infective endocarditis (**437**). Systemic emboli commonly occur and occasionally mycotic aneurysms develop (**438**). This patient had infective endocarditis involving the aortic valve and rapidly developed an aneurysm involving the popliteal artery, shown in this angiogram.

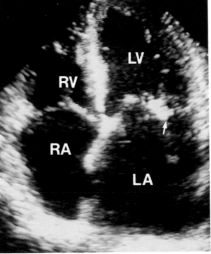

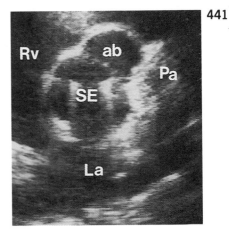

439-441 Cross-sectional echocardiography can be used to demonstrate vegetations or an aortic root abscess. Figure **439** (parasternal long axis view) shows aortic valve disease with a moderate-sized vegetation attached to the aortic valve (arrow). The floppy mitral valve is frequently the site of infective endocarditis; vegetations can occur both on the valve and on the ruptured chordae (arrow) as in this example (**440**). A complication of aortic valve endocarditis is aortic root abscess which can develop in spite of adequate antibiotic therapy and is an indication for early surgery. An abscess (ab) is seen lying anterior to the aortic root as a fluid filled space in a patient with a previous Starr-Edwards valve replacement (**441**).

INDEX

All references are to page numbers